NO GALLBLADDER DIET COOKBOOK

Post-Surgery Comfort Recipes: Healthy Eating Strategies for Low-Fat, Bile-Free Living

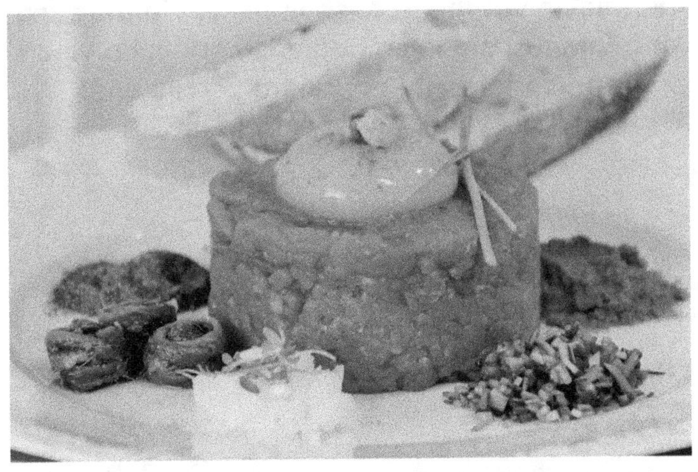

Thelma Howard

Table of Contents

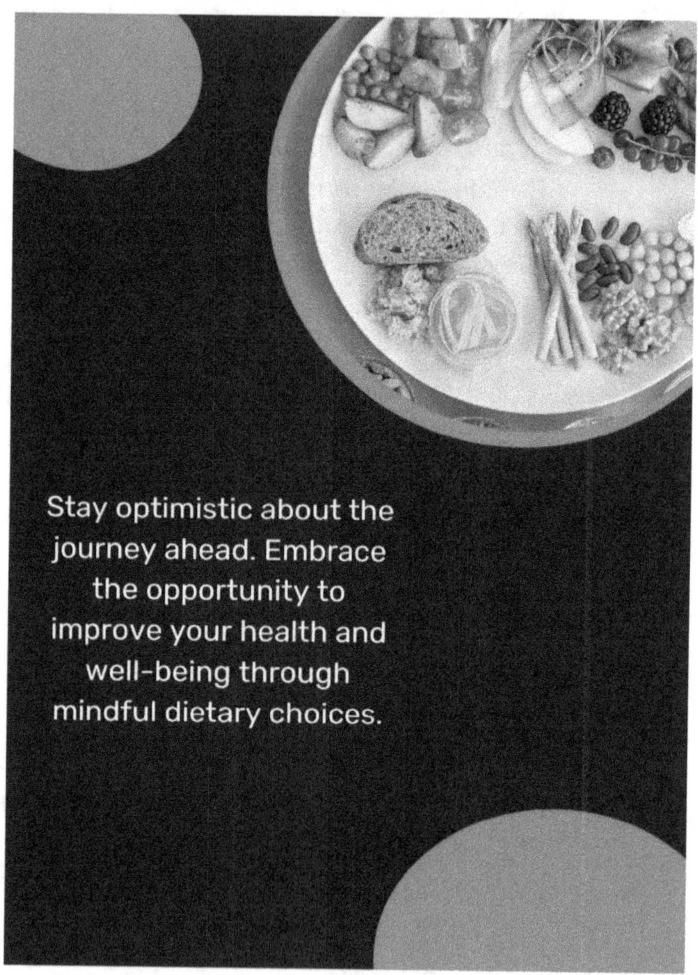

Stay optimistic about the journey ahead. Embrace the opportunity to improve your health and well-being through mindful dietary choices.

INTRODUCTION

Understanding the Role of the Gallbladder in Digestion

Located on the right side of the belly, beneath the liver, is a small, pear-shaped organ called the gallbladder. Despite its modest size, the gallbladder plays a crucial role in the process of digestion, particularly in the breakdown and absorption of fats.

Bile Production and Storage

One of the primary functions of the gallbladder is to store and concentrate bile, a digestive fluid produced by the liver. Bile is composed of water, bile salts, cholesterol, and waste products such as bilirubin. It is necessary for the small intestine to properly break down and absorb lipids.

Emulsification of Fats

When we consume fatty foods, bile is released from the gallbladder into the small intestine in response to the presence of fats. Bile emulsifies the fat molecules, breaking them down into smaller droplets. This process increases the surface area of the fat particles, making it easier for digestive enzymes to access and break them down further.

Facilitating Nutrient Absorption
In addition to aiding in fat digestion, bile also helps in the absorption of fat-soluble vitamins (A, D, E, and K) and other nutrients. By emulsifying fats, bile enables these nutrients to be absorbed through the intestinal lining and transported into the bloodstream for use by the body.

Regulation of Bile Secretion
The release of bile from the gallbladder is regulated by hormonal signals triggered by the presence of food, particularly fatty foods, in the digestive tract. Hormones such as cholecystokinin (CCK) stimulate the gallbladder to contract and release bile into the small intestine.

Gallbladder Removal and Digestive Implications
In cases where the gallbladder is removed due to disease or dysfunction (a procedure known as cholecystectomy), the ability to store and concentrate bile is compromised. As a result, bile is continuously secreted by the liver into the small intestine, but there is no longer a reservoir for its storage and concentration. This can lead to digestive issues, particularly with the digestion and absorption of fats.

Adapting to Life Without a Gallbladder
Individuals who have undergone gallbladder removal often need to make dietary modifications to manage their digestion effectively. This may include consuming smaller, more frequent meals, reducing

the intake of high-fat foods that can be difficult to digest, and incorporating dietary fiber to support healthy bowel function.

The gallbladder plays a vital role in the digestion and absorption of fats, as well as the regulation of nutrient uptake in the body. Understanding its functions can help individuals make informed dietary choices, especially following gallbladder removal, to support optimal digestion and overall well-being.

Life After Gallbladder Removal

Gallbladder removal, also known as cholecystectomy, is a common surgical procedure performed to alleviate symptoms associated with gallstones, gallbladder inflammation (cholecystitis), or other gallbladder-related conditions. While the removal of the gallbladder can provide relief from certain health issues, it also brings about changes in digestion and lifestyle that individuals should be aware of post-surgery.

Immediate Recovery
After gallbladder removal surgery, patients typically experience a period of recovery that may involve pain management, wound care, and dietary adjustments. Most patients can return home the same day or within a short hospital stay, but it may take several days to a few weeks to fully recover from the surgery.

Digestive Changes

One of the most significant changes after gallbladder removal is the alteration in the way the body processes and digests fats. Since the gallbladder is responsible for storing and concentrating bile, which aids in fat digestion, its removal can disrupt this process. Without the gallbladder, bile continuously drips into the small intestine, which can lead to difficulty digesting fatty foods, resulting in symptoms such as bloating, gas, diarrhea, or indigestion.

Dietary Modifications

To manage digestive issues and promote optimal digestion after gallbladder removal, individuals are often advised to make dietary modifications. This may include:

- Limiting the consumption of high-fat foods: Foods rich in saturated and trans fats, such as fried foods, fatty meats, creamy sauces, and processed snacks, can exacerbate digestive symptoms and ought to be avoided completely or consumed in moderation.
- Incorporating healthy fats: While some fats may be challenging to digest, others, such as those found in avocados, nuts, seeds, and fatty fish like salmon, provide essential nutrients and can be beneficial in small quantities.
- Eating smaller, more frequent meals: Eating smaller portions throughout the day can help

reduce the burden on the digestive system and minimize discomfort associated with larger meals.
- Increasing dietary fiber: Fiber-rich foods, such as fruits, vegetables, whole grains, and legumes, can help regulate bowel movements and promote digestive health.

Hydration and Fluid Intake

Staying hydrated is essential for maintaining digestive regularity and overall health, especially after gallbladder removal. Adequate fluid intake can help prevent constipation and promote the passage of stool through the digestive tract. Drinking water, herbal teas, and clear broths are good choices to stay hydrated.

Gradual Adjustment

It's important for individuals to understand that adjusting to life without a gallbladder may take time. Patience and experimentation with different foods and eating patterns are key to finding what works best for each person's unique digestive system. Keeping a food diary to track symptoms and identifying trigger foods can be helpful in managing post-cholecystectomy symptoms.

Consultation with Healthcare Providers

Individuals who have undergone gallbladder removal should maintain regular communication with their healthcare providers, including surgeons, gastroenterologists, and dietitians. These professionals can offer guidance, monitor progress, and address any concerns or complications that may arise during the postoperative period.

Life after gallbladder removal involves adapting to changes in digestion and lifestyle. By making informed dietary choices, staying hydrated, and seeking support from healthcare providers, individuals can effectively manage post-cholecystectomy symptoms and lead a healthy, fulfilling life.

Importance of Dietary Modifications

Dietary modifications play a crucial role in maintaining and improving overall health and well-being. Whether it's managing chronic conditions, preventing disease, or optimizing nutritional intake, adjusting one's diet can have profound effects on physical, mental, and emotional health. Here's a comprehensive overview of the importance of dietary modifications:

1. Managing Chronic Conditions
   - Many chronic conditions, such as diabetes, hypertension, cardiovascular disease, and gastrointestinal disorders, can be influenced by diet. Making strategic dietary changes, such as reducing sodium intake for hypertension or managing carbohydrate intake for diabetes, can

help control symptoms and improve health outcomes.

2. Preventing Disease

- A well-balanced diet rich in fruits, vegetables, whole grains, lean proteins, and healthy fats can help prevent various diseases and health conditions. For example, consuming a diet low in saturated fats and cholesterol can reduce the risk of developing heart disease, while a diet high in fiber can lower the risk of colorectal cancer.

3. Supporting Weight Management

- Dietary modifications are essential for achieving and maintaining a healthy weight. By controlling portion sizes, choosing nutrient-dense foods, and being mindful of calorie intake, individuals can effectively manage their weight and reduce the risk of obesity-related health issues, such as type 2 diabetes and joint problems.

4. Enhancing Nutritional Intake

- Dietary modifications can help ensure adequate intake of essential nutrients, vitamins, and minerals necessary for optimal health and functioning. By emphasizing a variety of nutrient-rich foods, individuals can meet their nutritional needs and support various bodily processes, including metabolism, immune function, and tissue repair.

5. **Managing Food Allergies and Intolerances**

- For individuals with food allergies or intolerances, dietary modifications are essential for avoiding trigger foods and preventing adverse reactions. Eliminating or reducing exposure to allergens and identifying suitable substitutes can help manage symptoms and improve quality of life.

6. **Improving Digestive Health**

- Diet plays a significant role in digestive health, influencing factors such as gut microbiota composition, bowel regularity, and gastrointestinal function. Dietary modifications, such as increasing fiber intake, staying hydrated, and avoiding trigger foods, can promote digestive comfort and reduce the risk of gastrointestinal disorders.

7. **Promoting Longevity and Vitality**

- Adopting a balanced and nutritious diet is associated with improved longevity and vitality. A diet rich in antioxidants, phytonutrients, and anti-inflammatory compounds can help protect against cellular damage, oxidative stress, and age-related diseases, contributing to a longer, healthier lifespan.

8. **Supporting Mental and Emotional Well-Being**

- Dietary modifications can impact mental and emotional health by influencing neurotransmitter function, mood regulation, and cognitive performance. Consuming a diet rich in omega-3 fatty acids, vitamins, and minerals can support brain health and emotional resilience, reducing the risk of depression, anxiety, and cognitive decline.

Dietary modifications are instrumental in promoting health, preventing disease, and enhancing overall well-being. By making informed choices about food and nutrition, individuals can optimize their health outcomes and enjoy a higher quality of life at every stage.

Adapting to the No Gallbladder Diet with Flavorful Meals Cookbook

Navigating life without a gallbladder can present dietary challenges, but with the right resources and guidance, individuals can adapt to their new dietary needs and continue to enjoy delicious and satisfying meals. The "No Gallbladder Diet Cookbook" is designed to support individuals in making the transition to a gallbladder-friendly diet while still savoring flavorful and nourishing dishes. Here's how this cookbook can help individuals adapt to the no gallbladder diet and enjoy tasty meals:

1. Education and Understanding
The cookbook provides essential information about the role of the gallbladder in digestion and explains the dietary modifications necessary after gallbladder removal. By understanding how certain

foods and ingredients can impact digestion, individuals can make informed choices when selecting recipes and planning meals.

2. Recipe Selection and Modification

The cookbook features a diverse selection of recipes tailored to the needs of individuals living without a gallbladder. From breakfast options to main courses, snacks, and desserts, each recipe is thoughtfully crafted to be low in fat, easy to digest, and packed with flavor. Recipes are also adaptable, allowing individuals to make modifications based on personal preferences and dietary restrictions.

3. Focus on Flavor and Variety

Despite dietary restrictions, the cookbook emphasizes flavor and variety, showcasing a range of ingredients, herbs, and spices that can enhance the taste of meals without compromising digestive health. Whether it's incorporating fresh herbs, citrus zest, or aromatic spices, each recipe is designed to tantalize the taste buds and make mealtime enjoyable.

4. Nutritional Balance and Wellness

The cookbook emphasizes the importance of maintaining nutritional balance and overall wellness while following a no gallbladder diet. Recipes are carefully curated to include nutrient-rich ingredients that support optimal health, such as lean proteins, whole grains, fruits, vegetables, and healthy fats. By focusing on wholesome and nourishing foods, individuals can feel confident in their dietary choices and promote overall well-being.

5. Practical Tips and Guidance

In addition to recipes, the cookbook provides practical tips and guidance for meal planning, grocery shopping, and dining out. Whether it's navigating restaurant menus, deciphering food labels, or stocking a pantry with gallbladder-friendly staples, individuals will find helpful strategies to make mealtime easier and more enjoyable.

6. Encouragement and Support

Living without a gallbladder can be challenging, but the cookbook offers encouragement and support to individuals as they adapt to their new dietary lifestyle. Through inspiring anecdotes, success stories, and motivational tips, individuals can feel empowered to take charge of their health and embrace the journey to better digestion and well-being.

The "No Gallbladder Diet Cookbook" serves as a valuable resource for individuals seeking to adapt to life without a gallbladder while still enjoying flavorful and satisfying meals. With its focus on education, recipe variety, nutritional balance, practical tips, and support, the cookbook empowers individuals to make the most of their dietary choices and thrive on their wellness journey.

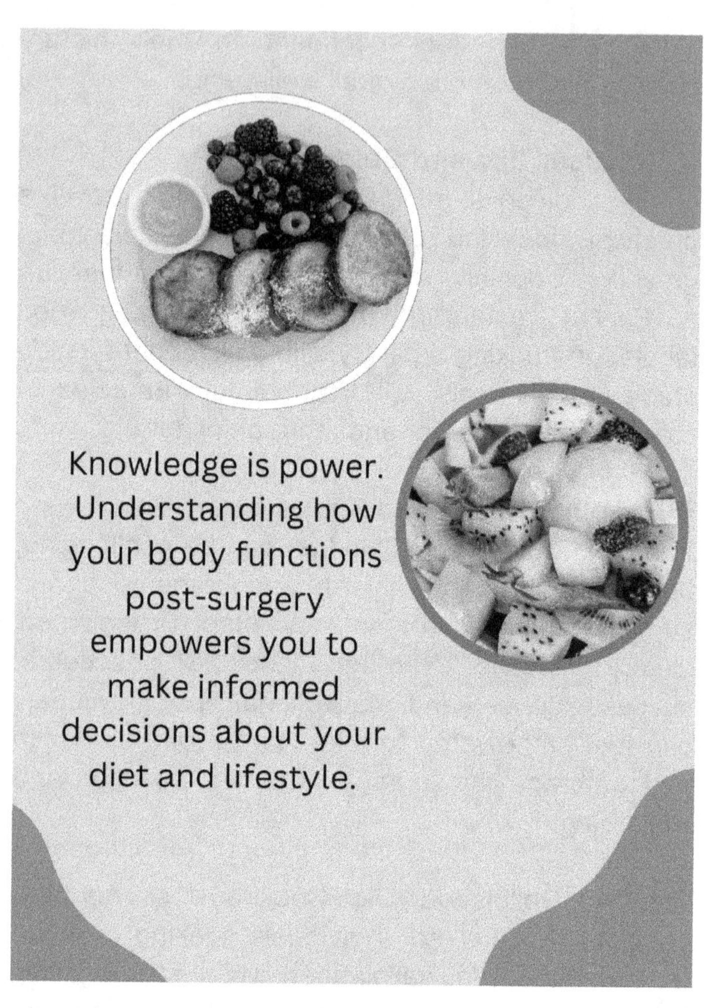

Knowledge is power.
Understanding how
your body functions
post-surgery
empowers you to
make informed
decisions about your
diet and lifestyle.

CHAPTER ONE

The Basics of a No Gallbladder Diet

Overview of Dietary Adjustments

Dietary adjustments are essential for promoting health, managing medical conditions, and addressing specific dietary needs. Whether it's adapting to a new lifestyle, managing chronic diseases, or optimizing nutritional intake, making informed dietary choices can have a profound impact on overall well-being. Here's a comprehensive overview of dietary adjustments:

1. Understanding Individual Needs

Dietary adjustments should be tailored to individual needs, taking into account factors such as age, gender, activity level, medical history, and personal preferences. What works for one person may not work for another, so it's important to consider individual circumstances when making dietary changes.

2. Identifying Dietary Goals

Before making dietary adjustments, it's important to identify specific goals and objectives. Whether it's achieving weight loss, managing blood sugar levels, reducing cholesterol, or improving digestive health, setting clear dietary goals can provide direction and motivation for making meaningful changes.

3. Assessing Current Dietary Patterns

Understanding current dietary habits and patterns is essential for identifying areas that may need adjustment. Keeping a food diary, tracking meals and snacks, and assessing nutrient intake can help individuals gain insight into their eating habits and identify areas for improvement.

4. Incorporating Nutrient-Rich Foods

Dietary adjustments should prioritize the inclusion of nutrient-rich foods that provide essential vitamins, minerals, antioxidants, and phytonutrients. Fruits, vegetables, whole grains, lean proteins, and healthy fats should form the foundation of a balanced diet, providing the body with the nutrients it needs for optimal functioning.

5. Limiting Processed Foods and Added Sugars

Processed foods, sugary snacks, and sweetened beverages should be limited or avoided as much as possible. These foods often contain added sugars, unhealthy fats, and artificial additives that can contribute to weight gain, inflammation, and chronic diseases such as diabetes and heart disease.

6. Moderating Portion Sizes

Portion control is an important aspect of dietary adjustments, especially for weight management and calorie control. Learning to recognize appropriate portion sizes and practicing mindful eating can help prevent overeating and promote a healthy balance of nutrients.

7. **Managing Macronutrient Intake** Balancing macronutrients—carbohydrates, proteins, and fats—is key to achieving a well-rounded diet. Emphasizing complex carbohydrates, lean proteins, and healthy fats can help stabilize blood sugar levels, support muscle growth and repair, and promote satiety and energy levels.

8. Staying Hydrated

Adequate hydration is essential for overall health and well-being. Drinking plenty of water throughout the day helps maintain proper hydration, supports digestion, regulates body temperature, and flushes out toxins and waste products.

9. Seeking Professional Guidance

For individuals with specific dietary needs or medical conditions, seeking guidance from a registered dietitian, nutritionist, or healthcare provider is recommended. These professionals can provide personalized dietary recommendations, address nutritional deficiencies, and offer support and guidance on making sustainable lifestyle changes.

Dietary adjustments are an integral part of promoting health, preventing disease, and optimizing nutritional intake. By understanding individual needs, setting clear goals, incorporating nutrient-rich foods, limiting processed foods, moderating portion sizes, and seeking professional guidance when needed, individuals can make meaningful dietary changes that support their overall well-being and vitality.

Recommended Foods and Beverages for a No Gallbladder Diet

Following the removal of the gallbladder (cholecystectomy), dietary adjustments become necessary to support digestion and minimize discomfort. The absence of the gallbladder affects the body's ability to process fats efficiently, making it important to choose foods and beverages that are gentle on the digestive system while still providing essential nutrients.

Here's a comprehensive overview of recommended foods and beverages for a no gallbladder diet:

1. Lean Proteins

Choose lean protein sources such as skinless poultry, fish, seafood, lean cuts of beef or pork, tofu, tempeh, and legumes. These options provide essential amino acids without the excess fat that can be difficult to digest.

2. Low-Fat Dairy

Opt for low-fat or fat-free dairy products such as skim milk, yogurt, cottage cheese, and low-fat cheese. These dairy options provide calcium and protein without the added burden of excess fat.

3. Whole Grains

Include whole grains such as brown rice, quinoa, oats, barley, whole wheat bread, and whole grain pasta in your diet. These foods are rich in fiber, vitamins, and minerals, and they can help support digestive health and regulate bowel movements.

4. Fruits and Vegetables

Choose a variety of colorful fruits and vegetables, including leafy greens, berries, apples, pears, bananas, carrots, bell peppers, and squash. These foods are rich in vitamins, minerals, antioxidants, and dietary fiber, which support overall health and digestion.

5. Healthy Fats

Incorporate sources of healthy fats such as avocados, nuts, seeds, olive oil, and fatty fish (e.g., salmon, mackerel, trout). These foods provide essential fatty acids and can be easier to digest compared to saturated and trans fats.

6. Cooked Vegetables

Cook vegetables to make them easier to digest, especially those that are high in insoluble fiber or contain tough skins and seeds. Steaming, sautéing, or roasting vegetables can help break down fibers and make them more tolerable for digestion.

7. High-Fiber Foods in Moderation

While fiber is important for digestive health, individuals with no gallbladder may need to moderate their intake of high-fiber foods initially. Gradually introduce fiber-rich foods such as whole grains, fruits, and vegetables into your diet to assess tolerance and prevent digestive discomfort.

8. Herbal Teas and Infusions

Enjoy herbal teas and infusions such as peppermint tea, ginger tea, chamomile tea, and fennel tea. These beverages can help soothe the digestive tract, alleviate gas and bloating, and promote overall digestive comfort.

9. Plenty of Water

Drink lots of water throughout the day to stay hydrated. Adequate hydration supports digestion, helps prevent constipation, and promotes overall health and well-being.

10. Small, Frequent Meals

Opt for smaller, more frequent meals throughout the day rather than large, heavy meals. Eating smaller portions helps reduce the workload on the digestive system and can minimize discomfort after eating.

A no gallbladder diet should focus on lean proteins, low-fat dairy, whole grains, fruits, vegetables, healthy fats, and plenty of water. By choosing foods and beverages that are gentle on the digestive system and incorporating them into balanced meals, individuals can support optimal digestion and overall well-being after gallbladder removal.

Foods to Avoid

Avoiding certain foods can be essential for managing health conditions, preventing discomfort, and promoting overall well-being.
Here's a comprehensive overview of foods to avoid:

1. High-Fat Foods

Foods high in saturated and trans fats can be challenging to digest, especially for individuals without a gallbladder. These include fatty cuts of meat, processed meats, full-fat dairy products, fried foods, and rich desserts.

2. Greasy or Fried Foods

Greasy and fried foods are heavy on the digestive system and can lead to discomfort, bloating, and indigestion. These foods include fried chicken, French fries, potato chips, and deep-fried snacks.

3. Spicy Foods

Spicy foods, particularly those containing hot peppers, chili powder, or spicy sauces, can irritate the digestive tract and exacerbate symptoms such as acid reflux, heartburn, and abdominal discomfort.

4. Rich Sauces and Creamy Dishes

Cream-based sauces, creamy soups, and rich gravies are often high in fat and can be difficult to digest, especially for individuals with compromised gallbladder function. These dishes should be consumed sparingly or avoided altogether.

5. Processed and Packaged Foods

Processed and packaged foods often contain additives, preservatives, and unhealthy fats that can disrupt digestion and contribute to inflammation. Examples include processed meats, canned soups, instant noodles, and packaged snacks.

6. High-Lactose Dairy Products

Dairy products high in lactose, such as whole milk, cream, ice cream, and soft cheeses, can be hard to digest, especially for individuals with lactose intolerance or compromised digestive function.

7. Carbonated Beverages

Carbonated beverages, including soda, sparkling water, and fizzy drinks, can cause gas and bloating in the digestive tract. These beverages also tend to be high in sugar or artificial sweeteners, which can negatively impact overall health.

8. Citrus Fruits and Juices

Citrus fruits and juices, such as oranges, grapefruits, lemons, and limes, are acidic and can aggravate acid reflux and digestive discomfort in some individuals. It's best to consume these foods in moderation or avoid them if they trigger symptoms.

9. High-Fiber Foods

While fiber is essential for digestive health, high-fiber foods can be difficult to digest for some individuals, especially in large quantities. Foods high in insoluble fiber, such as raw vegetables, whole grains, and certain fruits with skins or seeds, may need to be limited or cooked to make them easier to digest.

10. Alcohol and Caffeinated Beverages

Alcohol and caffeinated beverages, including coffee, tea, and energy drinks, can irritate the digestive tract and worsen symptoms such as acid reflux, heartburn, and stomach discomfort. Limiting or avoiding these beverages can help manage digestive issues and promote overall wellness.

Avoiding certain foods and beverages can help individuals manage digestive discomfort, prevent exacerbation of symptoms, and support overall digestive health. By making mindful choices and paying attention to how different foods affect their bodies, individuals can optimize their diets and enhance their well-being.

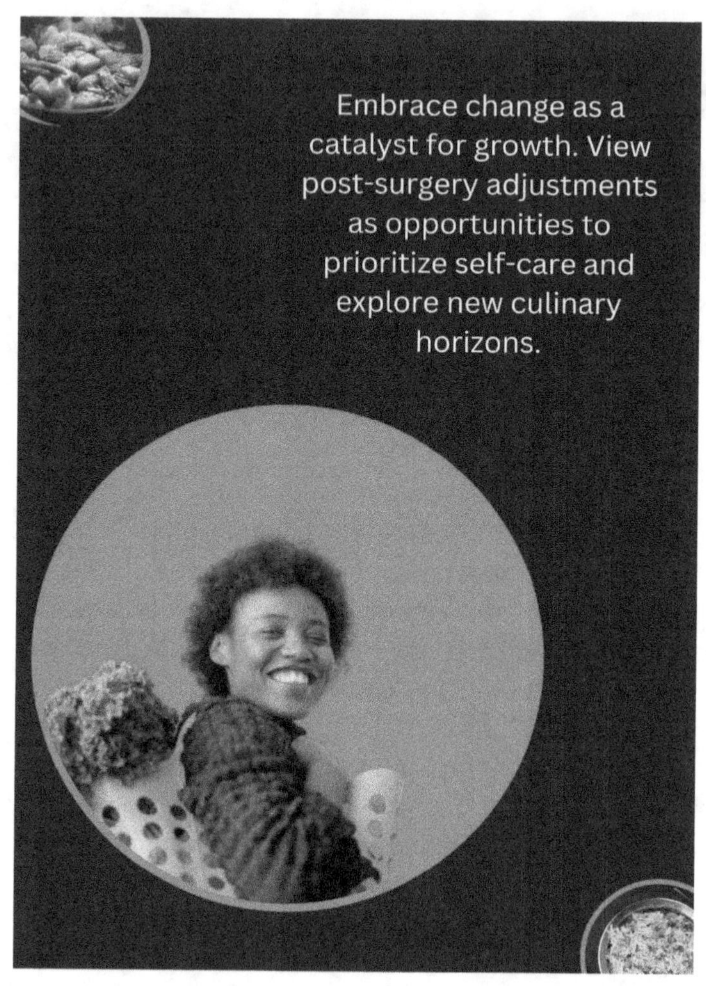
Embrace change as a
catalyst for growth. View
post-surgery adjustments
as opportunities to
prioritize self-care and
explore new culinary
horizons.

CHAPTER TWO

Essential Nutrients and Substitutions

Ensuring Nutritional Balance

Maintaining nutritional balance is particularly important for individuals following a no gallbladder diet. After gallbladder removal, the body's ability to process fats efficiently is compromised, necessitating dietary adjustments to support digestion and overall health. Achieving nutritional balance in a no gallbladder diet involves focusing on nutrient-dense foods, managing fat intake, and incorporating essential nutrients while minimizing digestive discomfort.

Here's a comprehensive guide to ensuring nutritional balance in a no gallbladder diet:

1. Prioritize Lean Proteins

Lean protein sources such as poultry, fish, seafood, tofu, tempeh, legumes, and low-fat dairy products should be prioritized in a no gallbladder diet. These options provide essential amino acids for muscle repair and growth without overloading the digestive system with excess fat.

2. Choose Healthy Fats Wisely

Opt for healthy fats such as olive oil, avocado oil, nuts, seeds, and fatty fish like salmon and trout. These fats contain omega-3 fatty acids, which support heart health and provide essential nutrients without causing digestive distress.

3. Include Fiber-Rich Foods

Incorporate fiber-rich foods such as fruits, vegetables, whole grains, legumes, and nuts into meals and snacks. Fiber promotes digestive health, regulates bowel movements, and helps maintain satiety, supporting overall well-being.

4. Moderate Fat Intake

While healthy fats are important, it's essential to moderate fat intake to avoid overwhelming the digestive system. Choose lean cuts of meat, trim visible fat from poultry, and limit fried and greasy foods to prevent discomfort after meals.

5. Emphasize Whole Foods

Whole foods, including fresh fruits, vegetables, whole grains, lean proteins, and healthy fats, should form the basis of a no gallbladder diet. These nutrient-dense foods provide essential vitamins, minerals, antioxidants, and fiber for optimal health.

6. Be Mindful of Portions

Pay attention to portion sizes to prevent overeating and minimize digestive discomfort. Eating smaller, more frequent meals throughout the day can help regulate blood sugar levels and support efficient digestion.

7. **Include Digestive Aids**

Incorporate digestive aids such as probiotic-rich foods (yogurt, kefir, sauerkraut) and digestive enzymes into the diet to support gut health and enhance digestion. These supplements can help alleviate digestive symptoms and improve nutrient absorption.

8. **Stay Hydrated**

Adequate hydration is essential for maintaining digestive health and overall well-being. Drink plenty of water throughout the day and consume hydrating foods such as fruits and vegetables to prevent dehydration and support digestive function.

9. **Monitor Symptoms**

Pay attention to how different foods affect digestive symptoms and adjust dietary choices accordingly. Keep a food diary to track meals, symptoms, and dietary patterns to identify triggers and make informed decisions about food choices.

10. **Seek Professional Guidance**

Consult with a registered dietitian or healthcare provider for personalized guidance and recommendations tailored to individual dietary needs and health goals. These professionals can provide valuable insight, support, and practical strategies for achieving nutritional balance in a no gallbladder diet.

Ensuring nutritional balance in a no gallbladder diet involves prioritizing lean proteins, choosing healthy fats, incorporating fiber-rich foods, moderating fat intake, emphasizing whole foods, being mindful of portions, including digestive aids, staying hydrated, monitoring symptoms, and seeking professional guidance. By following these principles, individuals can support digestive health, minimize discomfort, and optimize overall well-being on a no gallbladder diet.

Substitutes for High-Fat Ingredients

Maintaining a balanced diet after gallbladder removal involves minimizing the consumption of high-fat ingredients to prevent digestive discomfort and promote overall well-being. Incorporating substitutes for high-fat ingredients in recipes can help individuals follow a no gallbladder diet without sacrificing flavor or satisfaction. Here's a comprehensive guide to substitutes for high-fat ingredients in a no gallbladder diet:

1. Vegetable Broths and Stocks
Use vegetable broths or stocks as substitutes for fatty meat broths or stocks in soups, stews, and sauces. Vegetable broths add flavor and depth without the excess fat content.

2. Low-Fat Dairy Products
Substitute full-fat dairy products such as whole milk, cream, and cheese with low-fat or fat-free

options. Opt for skim milk, low-fat yogurt, cottage cheese, or reduced-fat cheese to reduce the overall fat content in recipes.

3. Greek Yogurt

Replace sour cream or mayonnaise with Greek yogurt in dips, dressings, and sauces. Greek yogurt provides a creamy texture and tangy flavor while offering protein and probiotics.

4. Applesauce or Mashed Bananas

Use unsweetened applesauce or mashed bananas as substitutes for oil or butter in baking recipes. These alternatives add moisture and sweetness to baked goods without the need for added fats.

5. Lean Protein Sources

Choose lean protein sources such as skinless poultry, fish, seafood, tofu, tempeh, and legumes instead of fatty cuts of meat. These options provide essential nutrients without the excess fat content.

6. Avocado Puree

Use mashed avocado as a substitute for butter or mayonnaise in spreads, sandwiches, and dips. Avocado provides heart-healthy fats and adds creaminess and richness to recipes.

7. Nutritional Yeast

Sprinkle nutritional yeast over popcorn, salads, or pasta dishes as a substitute for cheese.

Nutritional yeast adds a cheesy flavor without the saturated fat content of traditional cheese.

8. Citrus Juices and Vinegars

Use citrus juices (lemon, lime, orange) and vinegars (balsamic, apple cider) to add acidity and brightness to dishes without relying on high-fat ingredients. Citrus juices and vinegars enhance flavor while keeping fat content low.

9. Herbs and Spices

Enhance the flavor of dishes with herbs and spices such as garlic, onion, basil, oregano, paprika, cumin, and chili powder. Herbs and spices add depth and complexity to recipes without the need for added fats.

10. Toasted Nuts and Seeds

Incorporate toasted nuts and seeds as garnishes or toppings for salads, soups, and grain dishes. Toasted nuts and seeds provide crunch and flavor without contributing excessive amounts of fat.

By incorporating these substitutes for high-fat ingredients in a no gallbladder diet, individuals can enjoy flavorful and satisfying meals while supporting digestive health and overall well-being. Experimenting with different ingredients and cooking techniques can help individuals discover delicious and nutritious alternatives that align with their dietary goals.

Incorporating Fiber and Protein

A no gallbladder diet requires careful consideration of dietary choices to support digestion, manage symptoms, and maintain overall health. Incorporating adequate fiber and protein into meals is crucial for promoting satiety, regulating blood sugar levels, and supporting digestive health. Here's a comprehensive guide to incorporating fiber and protein in a no gallbladder diet:

1. High-Fiber Foods

Consume a diet high in fruits, vegetables, whole grains, legumes, nuts, and seeds, as well as other fiber-rich foods. These foods help promote regular bowel movements, prevent constipation, and support overall digestive health.

2. Whole Grains

Choose whole grains such as brown rice, quinoa, oats, barley, and whole wheat bread instead of refined grains. Whole grains provide fiber, vitamins, minerals, and antioxidants that contribute to digestive health and overall well-being.

3. Beans and Legumes

Incorporate beans, lentils, chickpeas, and other legumes into soups, stews, salads, and main dishes. Legumes are rich in fiber and protein, making them filling and satisfying additions to meals.

4. Fruits and Vegetables

Make it a point to eat a range of vibrant fruits and veggies. These foods are naturally high in fiber, vitamins, minerals, and antioxidants that support digestive health and immune function.

5. Leafy Greens

Include leafy greens such as spinach, kale, Swiss chard, and collard greens in salads, smoothies, soups, and stir-fries. Leafy greens are low in calories and high in fiber, making them excellent choices for promoting satiety and digestive health.

6. Lean Protein Sources

Choose lean protein sources such as skinless poultry, fish, seafood, tofu, tempeh, eggs, and low-fat dairy products. Lean proteins provide essential amino acids for muscle repair and growth without adding excess fat to the diet.

7. Greek Yogurt

Incorporate Greek yogurt into breakfasts, snacks, and desserts. Greek yogurt is high in protein and probiotics, which support digestive health and promote satiety.

8. Nuts and Seeds

Enjoy nuts and seeds as snacks or additions to salads, yogurt, and oatmeal. Nuts and seeds are rich in protein, healthy fats, fiber, vitamins, and minerals that contribute to overall health and well-being.

9. Protein Supplements

Consider incorporating protein supplements such as whey protein powder, pea protein powder, or collagen peptides into smoothies, shakes, or baked goods. Protein supplements can help increase protein intake and support muscle recovery and repair.

10. Balanced Meals

Aim to create balanced meals that include a combination of fiber-rich carbohydrates, lean proteins, healthy fats, and vegetables. Balanced meals help stabilize blood sugar levels, promote satiety, and support overall health and well-being.

By incorporating these strategies for increasing fiber and protein intake into a no gallbladder diet, individuals can support digestive health, manage symptoms, and maintain optimal nutrition. Experiment with different foods, recipes, and meal combinations to find what works best for your dietary needs and preferences.

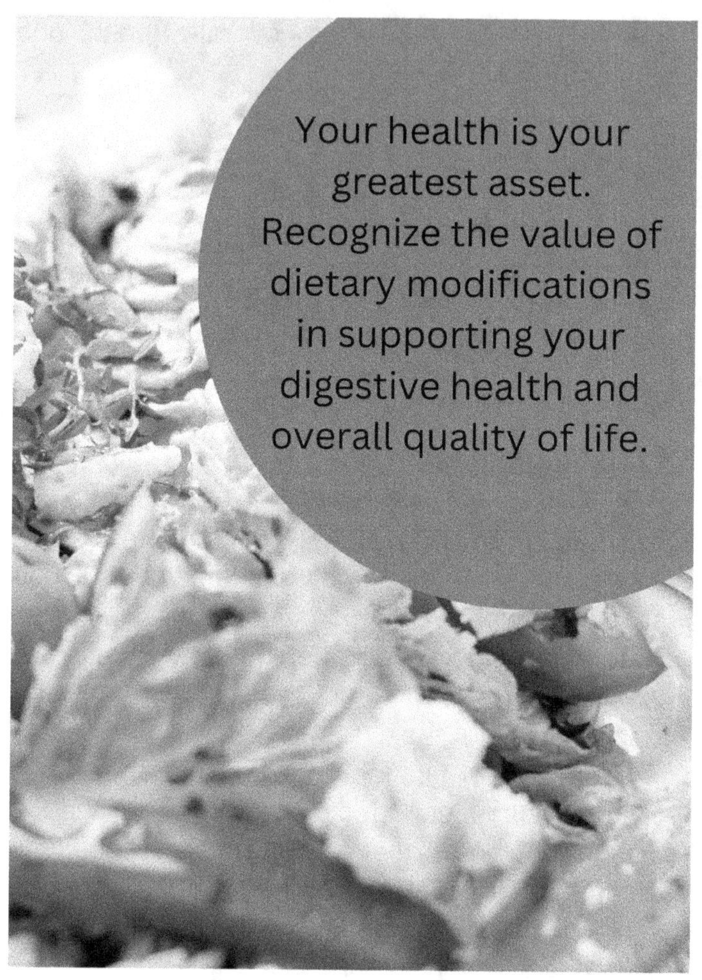
Your health is your greatest asset. Recognize the value of dietary modifications in supporting your digestive health and overall quality of life.

CHAPTER THREE

Meal Planning and Preparation

Strategies for Meal Preparation

Meal preparation is essential for individuals following a no gallbladder diet, as it allows for thoughtful planning and consideration of dietary choices to support digestion and overall well-being. By implementing effective meal preparation strategies, individuals can ensure they have nutritious and digestive-friendly meals readily available. Here are comprehensive strategies for meal preparation in a no gallbladder diet:

1. Plan Balanced Meals

Plan meals that include a balance of lean proteins, fiber-rich carbohydrates, healthy fats, and vegetables. Balanced meals help stabilize blood sugar levels and support digestive health.

2. Focus on Whole Foods

Prioritize whole foods such as fruits, vegetables, whole grains, lean proteins, and healthy fats in meal preparation. Whole foods provide essential nutrients and fiber while minimizing digestive discomfort.

3. Batch Cooking

Dedicate time each week to batch cook staple ingredients such as grains, beans, roasted vegetables, and lean proteins. Batch cooking saves time and ensures you have nutritious components readily available for assembling meals throughout the week.

4. Pre-cut Vegetables and Fruits

Wash, peel, and chop vegetables and fruits in advance to streamline meal preparation. Pre-cut produce can be stored in airtight containers in the refrigerator for easy access when preparing meals and snacks.

5. Choose Digestive-Friendly Ingredients

Select ingredients that are gentle on the digestive system, such as cooked vegetables, lean proteins, whole grains, and low-fat dairy products. Avoid high-fat, greasy, and heavily processed foods that may exacerbate digestive discomfort.

6. Portion Control

Use portion control containers or measuring cups to portion out ingredients and prevent overeating. Portion control promotes weight management objectives by regulating caloric intake.

7. Incorporate Meal Prep Containers

Invest in meal prep containers of various sizes to portion out meals and store leftovers. Meal prep containers make it easy to pack nutritious meals for work, school, or travel and prevent the need for last-minute meal decisions.

8. Experiment with One-Pot Meals

Prepare one-pot meals such as soups, stews, casseroles, and stir-fries that incorporate a variety of ingredients into a single dish. One-pot meals simplify meal preparation and minimize cleanup while offering a balanced combination of nutrients.

9. Include Make-Ahead Breakfasts

Prepare make-ahead breakfast options such as overnight oats, breakfast burritos, egg muffins, or chia seed pudding. Make-ahead breakfasts save time in the morning and ensure you start the day with a nutritious meal.

10. Freeze Meals for Later

Prepare extra portions of meals and freeze them in individual or family-sized portions for later use. Frozen meals provide convenient options for busy days and help reduce food waste.

11. Label and Date Meals

Label and date meal prep containers to keep track of the contents and ensure freshness. Proper labeling helps identify meals easily and prevents confusion about expiration dates.

12. Incorporate Variety

Keep meal preparation interesting by incorporating a variety of flavors, textures, and cuisines into your meals. Experiment with new recipes and ingredients to prevent monotony and promote enjoyment of meals.

By implementing these strategies for meal preparation, individuals following a no gallbladder diet can simplify the process of planning, cooking, and enjoying nutritious and digestive-friendly meals. Consistent meal preparation promotes adherence to dietary guidelines, supports digestive health, and contributes to overall well-being.

Weekly Meal Plans

Creating a weekly meal plan is an effective strategy for individuals following a no gallbladder diet to ensure they have nutritious and digestive-friendly meals throughout the week. A well-planned meal plan helps streamline grocery shopping, saves time in the kitchen, and promotes adherence to dietary guidelines.

Here's a comprehensive guide to creating weekly meal plans.

1. Assess Dietary Needs

Before creating a meal plan, assess your dietary needs, preferences, and any specific dietary restrictions or recommendations from your healthcare provider. Consider factors such as calorie requirements, macronutrient balance, and food sensitivities.

2. Plan Balanced Meals

Aim to include a balance of lean proteins, fiber-rich carbohydrates, healthy fats, and vegetables in each meal. Balanced meals help stabilize blood sugar levels, support digestion, and provide essential nutrients.

3. Include a Variety of Foods

Incorporate a variety of foods from different food groups to ensure you receive a wide range of nutrients and flavors. Experiment with different proteins, grains, vegetables, fruits, and herbs and spices to keep meals interesting and satisfying.

4. Batch Cooking Staples

Dedicate time at the beginning of the week to batch cook staple ingredients such as grains, beans, roasted vegetables, and lean proteins. Having these components prepared in advance makes meal assembly quicker and more convenient.

5. Rotate Protein Sources

Rotate protein sources throughout the week to incorporate variety and ensure you receive a diverse range of nutrients. Include options such as poultry, fish, seafood, tofu, tempeh, legumes, and eggs in your meal plan.

6. Plan for Digestive-Friendly Meals

Choose ingredients that are gentle on the digestive system, such as cooked vegetables, whole grains, lean proteins, and low-fat dairy products. Avoid high-fat, greasy, and heavily processed foods that may exacerbate digestive discomfort.

7. Incorporate Make-Ahead Options

Include make-ahead options for busy days or times when you may not have time to cook. Make-ahead breakfasts, lunches, and dinners such as overnight oats, salads in jars, and freezer-friendly casseroles can simplify mealtime.

8. Be Flexible

Be flexible with your meal plan and be open to making adjustments based on availability of ingredients, changes in schedule, or preferences. Use your meal plan as a guide rather than a rigid set of rules.

9. Plan for Leftovers

Plan meals that yield leftovers that can be enjoyed for lunch or dinner the following day. Leftovers can help minimize food waste and save time on meal preparation.

10. Consider Seasonal Produce

Take advantage of seasonal produce when planning your meals. Seasonal fruits and vegetables tend to be fresher, more flavorful, and more affordable, making them excellent choices for meal planning.

11. Include Snacks and Treats

Don't forget to plan for snacks and treats to enjoy throughout the week. Choose nutrient-dense snacks such as fruits, vegetables, nuts, and yogurt, and include occasional treats to satisfy cravings and prevent feelings of deprivation.

12. Review and Reflect

At the end of each week, review your meal plan and reflect on what worked well and what could be improved. Use feedback to refine your meal planning process and make adjustments for the following week.

By following these strategies for creating weekly meal plans, individuals following a no gallbladder diet can simplify meal preparation, support digestive health, and ensure they have nutritious and satisfying meals throughout the week. Consistent meal planning promotes adherence to dietary guidelines, reduces stress around mealtime, and contributes to overall well-being.

Tips for Dining Out and Traveling

Navigating dining out and traveling can pose challenges for individuals following a no gallbladder diet, as they need to be mindful of their food choices to prevent digestive discomfort and maintain overall well-being. However, with careful planning and awareness, dining out and traveling can still be enjoyable experiences. Here are comprehensive tips for dining out and traveling on a no gallbladder diet:

Dining Out

1. Research Restaurants in Advance

Before dining out, research restaurants in the area and look for options that offer a variety of dishes suitable for a no gallbladder diet. Check online menus or call ahead to inquire about menu options and modifications.

2. Choose Restaurants Wisely

Opt for restaurants that offer customizable dishes and accommodate special dietary needs. Look for establishments that prioritize fresh, whole ingredients and offer options such as grilled proteins, steamed vegetables, and salads with dressing on the side.

3. Communicate Dietary Restrictions

Inform your server about your dietary restrictions and ask for recommendations or modifications to suit your needs. Be specific about your requirements, such as avoiding fried foods, heavy sauces, or high-fat ingredients.

4. Customize Your Order

Don't hesitate to customize your order to meet your dietary preferences and restrictions. Ask for dressings, sauces, and condiments on the side, and request substitutions or modifications to dishes to make them more digestive-friendly.

5. Focus on Lean Proteins and Vegetables

Choose dishes that feature lean proteins such as grilled chicken, fish, or tofu, paired with steamed or sautéed vegetables. Avoid dishes that are deep-fried, breaded, or heavily sauced, as they may be harder to digest.

6. Be Mindful of Portions

Pay attention to portion sizes and avoid overeating, especially if you're dining at restaurants known for generous servings. Consider sharing a meal with a dining companion or asking for a half portion to control portion sizes.

7. Stay Hydrated

Drink plenty of water throughout the meal to aid digestion and prevent dehydration. Limit alcoholic beverages and sugary drinks, which can exacerbate digestive discomfort.

8. Practice Mindful Eating

Eat slowly, savoring each bite, and pay attention to hunger and fullness cues. Rather than waiting until you're quite full, stop eating when you feel content.

Traveling

1. Pack Snacks

Pack portable snacks such as nuts, seeds, dried fruits, whole grain crackers, and protein bars to have on hand while traveling. Having snacks readily available can help prevent hunger and avoid unhealthy food choices.

2. Research Dining Options

Research dining options at your destination and look for restaurants, grocery stores, or markets that offer nutritious and digestive-friendly choices. Consider booking accommodations with kitchenettes to prepare your own meals if necessary.

3. Bring Digestive Aids

Pack digestive aids such as probiotics, digestive enzymes, and over-the-counter medications to help manage digestive symptoms while traveling. These supplements can provide relief and support digestive health during your trip.

4. Stay Hydrated

Drink plenty of water while traveling to stay hydrated and support digestion. Carry a refillable water bottle and aim to drink water regularly throughout the day, especially in hot or dry climates.

5. Be Prepared for Flights:m

If you're flying, plan ahead for meals and snacks during the flight. Bring nutritious snacks and meals that are easy to transport and won't spoil, such as sandwiches, salads, fruits, and nuts.

6. Choose Smart Options

When dining out while traveling, choose restaurants that offer lighter fare options such as salads, grilled proteins, and vegetable-based dishes. Ask for modifications or substitutions to accommodate your dietary needs.

7. Listen to Your Body

Pay attention to how your body responds to different foods while traveling and adjust your choices accordingly. Be mindful of any symptoms or discomfort and make choices that support your digestive health and overall well-being.

By following these tips for dining out and traveling on a no gallbladder diet, individuals can make informed choices, manage digestive symptoms, and enjoy their culinary experiences while away from home. Planning ahead, communicating dietary needs, and prioritizing digestive-friendly options can help make dining out and traveling enjoyable and stress-free.

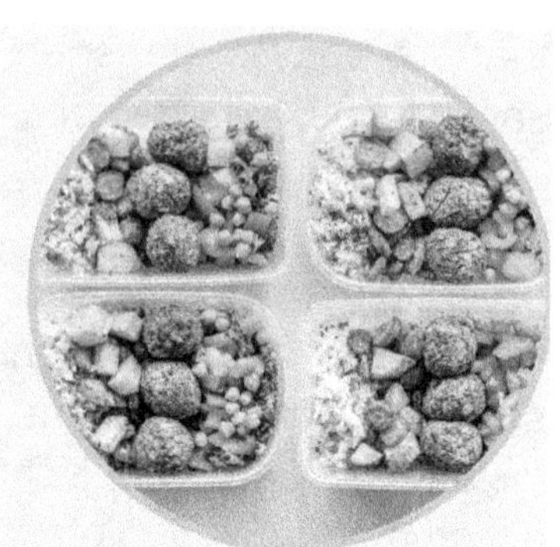

Nourish your body with wholesome ingredients that support vitality and well-being. Embrace the abundance of delicious and nutritious foods available to you.

CHAPTER FOUR

Breakfast Recipes

Low-Fat Breakfast Ideas

Scrambled Egg Whites with Spinach and Tomatoes
Ingredients:
- 4 egg whites
- 1 cup fresh spinach leaves, washed and chopped
- 1/2 cup cherry tomatoes, halved
- Salt and pepper to taste
- 1 teaspoon olive oil (optional)

Preparation Method:
1. Heat a non-stick skillet over medium heat. If using olive oil, add it to the skillet and spread it evenly.
2. In a bowl, whisk the egg whites until frothy. Adjust the amount of salt and pepper to taste.
3. Pour the egg whites into the skillet and let them cook for a minute or two until they begin to set.
4. Add the chopped spinach and halved cherry tomatoes to the skillet, distributing them evenly over the eggs.
5. Gently stir the mixture occasionally until the egg whites are fully cooked and the spinach is wilted.
6. Once cooked, transfer the scrambled egg whites with spinach and tomatoes to a serving plate.
7. Serve hot and enjoy.

Oatmeal Topped with Sliced Bananas and Almonds

Ingredients:
- 1/2 cup rolled oats
- 1 cup water or milk (almond milk, soy milk, or regular milk)
- 1 ripe banana, sliced
- 2 tablespoons sliced almonds
- Honey or maple syrup for drizzling (optional)
- Cinnamon (optional)

Preparation Method:
1. In a small saucepan, bring the water or milk to a boil.
2. Stir in the rolled oats and reduce the heat to low. Allow the oats to simmer for about 5 minutes, stirring occasionally, until they reach your desired consistency.
3. Once the oats are cooked, remove the saucepan from the heat and transfer the oatmeal to a serving bowl.
4. Arrange the sliced bananas on top of the oatmeal.
5. Sprinkle the sliced almonds over the bananas.
6. If desired, drizzle honey or maple syrup over the oatmeal for added sweetness.
7. Optional: Sprinkle with cinnamon for extra flavor.
8. Serve warm and enjoy your delicious oatmeal topped with sliced bananas and almonds.

Greek Yogurt Parfait with Berries and Granola
Ingredients:
- One cup of plain or flavored Greek yogurt
- 1/2 cup mixed berries (strawberries, blueberries, raspberries)
- 1/4 cup granola (homemade or store-bought)
- Honey or maple syrup for drizzling (optional)

Preparation Method:
1. In a serving glass or bowl, layer half of the Greek yogurt at the bottom.
2. Add half of the mixed berries on top of the yogurt layer.
3. Sprinkle half of the granola over the berries.
4. Repeat the layers with the remaining Greek yogurt, mixed berries, and granola.
5. If desired, drizzle honey or maple syrup over the top of the parfait for added sweetness.
6. Serve immediately as a nutritious breakfast or snack option.
7. Enjoy your Greek yogurt parfait with berries and granola.

Whole Grain Toast with Avocado Spread and Sliced Cucumbers

Ingredients:
- 2 slices of whole grain bread
- 1 ripe avocado
- 1 small cucumber, thinly sliced
- Salt and pepper to taste

- Optional: lemon juice, red pepper flakes, or garlic powder for additional flavor

Preparation Method:
1. Toast the slices of whole grain bread until golden brown and crispy.
2. While the bread is toasting, prepare the avocado spread. Cut the ripe avocado in half, remove the pit, and scoop the flesh into a small bowl.
3. Mash the avocado with a fork until smooth and creamy. Add salt, pepper, and any additional flavorings like lemon juice, red pepper flakes, or garlic powder to taste.
4. Once the toast is ready, spread the mashed avocado evenly over each slice.
5. Top the avocado spread with thinly sliced cucumbers, distributing them evenly.
6. Sprinkle with a little extra salt and pepper if desired.
7. Serve immediately and enjoy your delicious whole grain toast with avocado spread and sliced cucumbers.

Cottage Cheese Topped with Pineapple Chunks and Chia Seeds

Ingredients:
- 1 cup cottage cheese
- 1/2 cup pineapple chunks (fresh or canned, drained)
- 1 tablespoon chia seeds

- Honey or maple syrup are optional but add sweetness.

Preparation Method:

1. In a serving bowl, spoon the cottage cheese to create a base layer.
2. Top the cottage cheese with pineapple chunks, spreading them evenly over the surface.
3. Sprinkle chia seeds over the pineapple and cottage cheese.
4. Drizzle with honey or maple syrup if desired for added sweetness.
5. Serve immediately as a nutritious and satisfying snack or breakfast option.
6. Enjoy your cottage cheese topped with pineapple chunks and chia seeds.

Smoothie Made with Spinach, Banana, Almond Milk, and Protein Powder

Ingredients:

- 1 ripe banana, peeled and sliced
- 1 cup fresh spinach leaves, washed
- 1 cup unsweetened almond milk
- One scoop of unflavored or vanilla protein powder
- Optional: honey or maple syrup for sweetness, ice cubes for a colder smoothie

Preparation Method:

1. Place the sliced banana, fresh spinach leaves, almond milk, and protein powder in a blender.
2. If desired, add honey or maple syrup for sweetness, and ice cubes for a colder smoothie.

3. Blend all the ingredients until smooth and creamy, scraping down the sides of the blender if necessary.
4. Taste the smoothie and adjust sweetness or thickness by adding more honey, maple syrup, or almond milk if needed.
5. Once the desired consistency is reached, pour the smoothie into glasses.
6. Serve immediately as a nutritious and refreshing breakfast or snack option.
7. Enjoy your delicious smoothie made with spinach, banana, almond milk, and protein powder.

Veggie Omelet with Mushrooms, Bell Peppers, and Onions

Ingredients:
- 3 large eggs
- 1/4 cup sliced mushrooms
- 1/4 cup of bell peppers, chopped, any color.
- 1/4 cup diced onions
- Salt and pepper to taste
- One tablespoon cooking spray or olive oil.

Preparation Method:
1. In a small bowl, beat the eggs until well combined. Adjust the amount of salt and pepper to taste.
2. Heat olive oil or cooking spray in a non-stick skillet over medium heat.
3. Add the sliced mushrooms, diced bell peppers, and diced onions to the skillet. Cook until vegetables are tender, about 3-4 minutes.

4. Pour the beaten eggs evenly over the cooked vegetables in the skillet.

5. Allow the eggs to cook undisturbed for a few minutes until the edges start to set.

6. Gently lift the edges of the omelet with a spatula and tilt the skillet to let the uncooked eggs flow to the edges.

7. Once the omelet is mostly set but still slightly runny on top, fold it in half using the spatula.

8. Cook for another minute or until the eggs are fully set and cooked through.

9. Slide the omelet onto a plate and serve hot.

10. Enjoy your delicious veggie omelet with mushrooms, bell peppers, and onions.

Ingredients:

- 1/2 cup quinoa, rinsed
- 1 cup water
- One cup of unsweetened almond milk or any other type of milk.
- 1 apple, peeled and diced
- 1/2 teaspoon ground cinnamon
- Honey or maple syrup are optional but add sweetness.

Preparation Method:

1. In a medium saucepan, combine quinoa, water, and almond milk.

2. Heat the mixture on medium-high and bring it to a boil.

3. Reduce the heat to low, cover, and simmer for about 15-20 minutes, or until the quinoa is cooked and the liquid is absorbed.

4. To keep things from sticking and burning, stir periodically.

5. Once the quinoa is cooked, remove the saucepan from the heat.

6. Stir in the diced apples and ground cinnamon.

7. If desired, add honey or maple syrup for sweetness.

8. Serve the quinoa porridge warm in bowls.

9. Enjoy your comforting quinoa porridge with diced apples and cinnamon.

Low-Fat Cheese Quesadilla with Salsa and Black Beans

Ingredients:
- 2 whole wheat tortillas
- 1/2 cup low-fat shredded cheese (cheddar, mozzarella, or Mexican blend)
- 1/4 cup salsa
- 1/4 cup canned black beans, drained and rinsed
- Cooking spray or olive oil for greasing the skillet

Preparation Method:
1. Heat a non-stick skillet over medium heat.

2. Place one whole wheat tortilla in the skillet.

3. Sprinkle half of the shredded cheese evenly over the tortilla.

4. Top the cheese with black beans and salsa.

5. Sprinkle the remaining cheese over the salsa and black beans.

6. Place the second tortilla on top to cover the filling.

7. Cook the quesadilla for 2-3 minutes on each side, or until the tortillas are golden brown and the cheese is melted.

8. Carefully flip the quesadilla using a spatula and cook the other side until golden brown and cheese is melted.

9. Once cooked, transfer the quesadilla to a cutting board and let it cool for a minute.

10. Using a sharp knife, cut the quesadilla into wedge shapes.

11. Serve hot with additional salsa on the side, if desired.

12. Enjoy your tasty low-fat cheese quesadilla with salsa and black beans.

Buckwheat Pancakes with Fresh Fruit and a Drizzle of Honey

Ingredients:
- 1 cup buckwheat flour
- 1 tablespoon baking powder
- 1/4 teaspoon salt
- 1 tablespoon honey (plus extra for drizzling)
- 1 cup almond milk or any milk of your choice
- 1 large egg
- Cooking spray or oil for greasing the skillet
- Fresh fruit for topping (such as berries, bananas, or sliced peaches)

Preparation Method:
1. In a mixing bowl, whisk together the buckwheat flour, baking powder, and salt.

2. In another bowl, whisk together the honey, almond milk, and egg until well combined.

3. Mixing until just mixed, pour the wet components into the dry ingredients. Avoid over-mixing; some lumps are OK.

4. Heat a non-stick skillet or griddle over medium heat and lightly coat with cooking spray or oil.

5. Pour about 1/4 cup of batter onto the skillet for each pancake. Simmer for two to three minutes, or until surface bubbles appear and the edges appear firm.

6. After flipping the pancakes, heat for a further one to two minutes, or until they are cooked through and golden brown.

7. Remove the pancakes from the skillet and stack them on a plate.

8. Top the pancakes with fresh fruit of your choice and drizzle with honey.

9. Serve warm and enjoy your delicious buckwheat pancakes with fresh fruit and honey.

Egg Muffins with Spinach, Mushrooms, and Feta Cheese

Ingredients:
- 6 large eggs
- 1 cup fresh spinach, chopped
- 1/2 cup mushrooms, diced
- 1/4 cup crumbled feta cheese
- Salt and pepper to taste
- Oil or cooking spray to grease the muffin pan.

Preparation Method:

1. Preheat the oven to 350°F (175°C). Spray cooking oil or cooking spray into a muffin tin.

2. In a mixing bowl, crack the eggs and whisk them together until well beaten.

3. Stir in the chopped spinach, diced mushrooms, and crumbled feta cheese. Season with salt and pepper to taste.

4. Divide the egg mixture evenly among the muffin cups, filling each about 3/4 full.

5. Bake in the preheated oven for 18-20 minutes, or until the egg muffins are set and slightly golden on top.

6. Remove from the oven and allow the egg muffins to cool in the muffin tin for a few minutes.

7. Carefully remove the egg muffins from the muffin tin and transfer them to a wire rack to cool completely.

8. Once cooled, store the egg muffins in an airtight container in the refrigerator for up to 3-4 days.

9. Reheat in the microwave or enjoy them cold as a nutritious snack or breakfast option.

Low-Fat Yogurt Bowl with Sliced Peaches and Almonds

Ingredients:

- 1 cup low-fat yogurt (plain or flavored)
- 1 ripe peach, sliced
- 2 tablespoons sliced almonds
- Honey or maple syrup are optional but add sweetness.

Preparation Method:
1. In a serving bowl, spoon the low-fat yogurt to create a base layer.
2. Arrange the sliced peaches on top of the yogurt layer.
3. Sprinkle sliced almonds over the peaches.
4. If desired, drizzle honey or maple syrup over the yogurt bowl for added sweetness.
5. Serve immediately as a nutritious and satisfying snack or breakfast option.
6. Enjoy your low-fat yogurt bowl with sliced peaches and almonds.

Whole Grain Waffles with Greek Yogurt and Mixed Berries

Ingredients:
- 1 cup whole grain waffle mix
- 1/2 cup water or milk (almond milk, soy milk, or regular milk)
- Oil or cooking spray to grease the waffle iron.
- 1/2 cup Greek yogurt (plain or flavored)
- 1/2 cup mixed berries (strawberries, blueberries, raspberries)

Preparation Method:
1. As directed by the manufacturer, preheat your waffle iron.
2. In a mixing bowl, combine the whole grain waffle mix and water or milk. Stir until well combined and smooth.
3. Lightly grease the preheated waffle iron with cooking spray or oil.

4. Pour the waffle batter onto the center of the waffle iron, spreading it evenly.
5. Close the waffle iron and cook the waffle according to the manufacturer's instructions, until golden brown and crispy.
6. Once cooked, carefully remove the waffle from the iron and place it on a serving plate.
7. Top the waffle with Greek yogurt and mixed berries.
8. Serve immediately and enjoy your nutritious whole grain waffles with Greek yogurt and mixed berries.

Wrapped on a whole wheat tortilla, a breakfast burrito with scrambled eggs, black beans, and salsa

Ingredients:
- 2 large eggs, beaten
- 1/4 cup canned black beans, drained and rinsed
- 2 tablespoons salsa
- 1 whole wheat tortilla
- Salt and pepper to taste
- Cooking spray or oil for cooking

Preparation Method:
1. Heat a non-stick skillet over medium heat and lightly grease it with cooking spray or oil.
2. Pour the beaten eggs into the skillet and scramble them until cooked through.
3. To taste, add salt and pepper to the scrambled eggs.

4. Warm the black beans in the microwave or on the stove.
5. Heat the whole wheat tortilla in the microwave or on a skillet until warm and pliable.
6. Place the scrambled eggs and black beans in the center of the tortilla.
7. Top with salsa.
8. Fold in the sides of the tortilla and roll it up tightly to form a burrito.
9. Serve immediately and enjoy your delicious breakfast burrito with scrambled eggs, black beans, and salsa.

Chia Seed Pudding Topped with Sliced Strawberries and Shredded Coconut

Ingredients:
- 1/4 cup chia seeds
- 1 cup almond milk or any milk of your choice
- One tablespoon of maple syrup or honey (optional).
- 1/2 teaspoon vanilla extract
- 4-6 fresh strawberries, sliced
- 2 tablespoons shredded coconut

Preparation Method:
1. In a mixing bowl, combine the chia seeds, almond milk, honey or maple syrup (if using), and vanilla extract. Stir until well combined.
2. Cover the bowl and refrigerate the chia seed mixture for at least 2 hours or overnight, allowing it to thicken and set into a pudding-like consistency.

3. Once the chia seed pudding is set, give it a good stir.
4. Spoon the chia seed pudding into serving bowls or glasses.
5. Top the pudding with sliced strawberries and shredded coconut.
6. Serve chilled and enjoy your delightful chia seed pudding topped with sliced strawberries and shredded coconut.

Turkey Bacon and Egg Wrap with Spinach and Tomatoes
Ingredients:
- 2 slices of turkey bacon
- 2 large eggs
- 1 whole wheat tortilla
- 1/2 cup fresh spinach leaves
- 1/4 cup cherry tomatoes, sliced
- Salt and pepper to taste
- Cooking spray or oil for cooking

Preparation Method:
1. Heat a non-stick skillet over medium heat and lightly grease it with cooking spray or oil.
2. Cook the turkey bacon slices in the skillet until crispy, according to package instructions. Remove and set aside.
3. In the same skillet, crack the eggs and cook them to your desired doneness (scrambled, fried, or poached). Season with salt and pepper to taste.

4. While the eggs are cooking, warm the whole wheat tortilla in the microwave or on a skillet until pliable.

5. Place the cooked turkey bacon slices, scrambled eggs, fresh spinach leaves, and sliced cherry tomatoes in the center of the tortilla.

6. Fold in the sides of the tortilla and roll it up tightly to form a wrap.

7. Serve immediately and enjoy your delicious turkey bacon and egg wrap with spinach and tomatoes.

Brown Rice Congee with Poached Egg and Green Onions

Ingredients:
- 1/2 cup brown rice
- 4 cups water or chicken broth
- 1 poached egg
- 2 green onions, thinly sliced
- Salt and pepper to taste
- Optional: soy sauce or sesame oil for added flavor

Preparation Method:
1. Till the water runs clear, rinse the brown rice under cold water.

2. In a large pot, bring the water or chicken broth to a boil over medium-high heat.

3. Add the rinsed brown rice to the pot and reduce the heat to low. Simmer, covered, for about 40-45 minutes, stirring occasionally, until the rice is soft and the congee is creamy.

4. Once the congee reaches your desired consistency, season with salt and pepper to taste.

5. Ladle the brown rice congee into serving bowls.

6. Top each bowl with a poached egg and sprinkle with sliced green onions.

7. Optional: Drizzle with soy sauce or sesame oil for added flavor.

8. Serve hot and enjoy your comforting brown rice congee with poached egg and green onions.

Breakfast Smoothie Bowl Topped with Sliced Kiwi, Coconut Flakes, and Pumpkin Seeds

Ingredients:
- 1 ripe banana, peeled and sliced
- 1 cup fresh spinach leaves
- 1/2 cup almond milk or any milk of your choice
- One scoop of unflavored or vanilla protein powder.
- Toppings: sliced kiwi, coconut flakes, pumpkin seeds

Preparation Method:

1. In a blender, combine the sliced banana, fresh spinach leaves, almond milk, and protein powder.

2. Blend until smooth and creamy, adding more milk if needed to reach your desired consistency.

3. Pour the smoothie into a bowl.

4. Arrange the sliced kiwi, coconut flakes, and pumpkin seeds on top of the smoothie bowl.

5. Serve immediately and enjoy your nutritious breakfast smoothie bowl topped with sliced kiwi, coconut flakes, and pumpkin seeds.

Baked Oatmeal Cups with Blueberries and Walnuts

Ingredients:
- 2 cups rolled oats
- 1 teaspoon baking powder
- 1/2 teaspoon ground cinnamon
- 1/4 teaspoon salt
- 1 large egg
- 1/4 cup honey or maple syrup
- 1 cup almond milk or any milk of your choice
- 1 teaspoon vanilla extract
- 1/2 cup fresh blueberries
- 1/4 cup chopped walnuts

Preparation Method:
1. Preheat your oven to 350°F (175°C) and grease a muffin tin with cooking spray or line it with muffin liners.
2. In a large mixing bowl, combine the rolled oats, baking powder, cinnamon, and salt.
3. In another bowl, whisk together the egg, honey or maple syrup, almond milk, and vanilla extract.
4. After adding the wet ingredients to the dry ingredients, thoroughly mix them together.
5. Gently mix in the chopped walnuts and blueberries.
6. Divide the oatmeal mixture evenly among the prepared muffin cups.
7. Bake in the preheated oven for 25-30 minutes, or until the oatmeal cups are set and golden brown on top.

8. Remove from the oven and let cool in the muffin tin for a few minutes before transferring to a wire rack to cool completely.

9. Once cooled, store the oatmeal cups in an airtight container in the refrigerator for up to one week.

10. Enjoy your delicious baked oatmeal cups with blueberries and walnuts for a nutritious breakfast or snack.

Whole Grain English Muffin with Almond Butter and Sliced Bananas

Ingredients:

-One English muffin with whole grains, divided and toasted.

- 2 tablespoons almond butter

- 1 ripe banana, sliced

Preparation Method:

1. Toast the whole grain English muffin halves until golden brown and crispy.

2. Spread 1 tablespoon of almond butter on each English muffin half.

3. Arrange the sliced bananas on top of the almond butter.

4. Serve immediately and enjoy your wholesome whole grain English muffin with almond butter and sliced bananas.

Veggie and Tofu Scramble with Zucchini, Kale, and Bell Peppers
Ingredients:
- 1/2 block extra-firm tofu, drained and crumbled
- 1 tablespoon olive oil
- 1 small zucchini, diced
- 1 cup kale leaves, chopped
- 1/2 bell pepper, diced
- Salt and pepper to taste
- Optional: nutritional yeast, turmeric, garlic powder for seasoning

Preparation Method:
1. In a skillet over medium heat, warm the olive oil.
2. Add the diced zucchini, chopped kale, and diced bell pepper to the skillet. Cook until vegetables are tender, about 5-7 minutes.
3. Add the crumbled tofu to the skillet and cook for another 3-5 minutes, stirring occasionally.
4. Season with salt, pepper, and any additional seasonings like nutritional yeast, turmeric, or garlic powder, according to taste.
5. Cook until the tofu is heated through and slightly golden.
6. Remove from heat and serve hot.
7. Enjoy your flavorful veggie and tofu scramble with zucchini, kale, and bell peppers as a nutritious breakfast option.

Low-Fat Yogurt Parfait with Mango Chunks and Toasted Coconut Flakes
Ingredients:
- 1 cup low-fat yogurt (plain or flavored)
- 1 ripe mango, peeled and diced
- 2 tablespoons toasted coconut flakes

Preparation Method:
1. In a serving glass or bowl, spoon a layer of low-fat yogurt.
2. Add a layer of diced mango chunks on top of the yogurt.
3. Repeat the layers with yogurt and mango until the glass or bowl is filled.
4. Top the parfait with toasted coconut flakes.
5. Serve immediately as a refreshing and nutritious breakfast or snack option.
6. Enjoy your delicious low-fat yogurt parfait with mango chunks and toasted coconut flakes.

Cottage Cheese Pancakes with Raspberry Compote
Ingredients for Pancakes:
- 1 cup cottage cheese
- 4 large eggs
- 1/2 cup rolled oats
- 1 teaspoon vanilla extract
- Cooking spray or oil for greasing the skillet

Ingredients for Raspberry Compote:
- 1 cup fresh or frozen raspberries
- 2 tablespoons water

- One tablespoon of maple syrup or honey (optional).

Preparation Method:
For Pancakes:
1. In a blender, combine cottage cheese, eggs, rolled oats, and vanilla extract. Blend until smooth.
2. Heat a non-stick skillet or griddle over medium heat and lightly grease it with cooking spray or oil.
3. Pour about 1/4 cup of batter onto the skillet for each pancake.
4. Cook until bubbles form on the surface of the pancake and the edges look set, about 2-3 minutes.
5. Flip the pancake and cook for an additional 1-2 minutes, or until golden brown and cooked through.
6. Repeat with the remaining batter.
7. Keep pancakes warm while you prepare the raspberry compote.

For Raspberry Compote:
1. In a small saucepan, combine raspberries, water, and honey or maple syrup (if using).
2. Over medium heat, bring the mixture to a simmer.
3. Cook, stirring occasionally, until the raspberries break down and the mixture thickens slightly, about 5-7 minutes.
4. Take off the heat and allow to cool a little.
5. Serve the cottage cheese pancakes topped with raspberry compote.

6. Enjoy your tasty cottage cheese pancakes with raspberry compote as a delightful breakfast treat.

Spinach and Feta Frittata with Cherry Tomatoes
Ingredients:
- 6 large eggs
- 1/4 cup milk (almond milk, soy milk, or regular milk)
- 2 cups fresh spinach leaves, washed
- 1/2 cup crumbled feta cheese
- 1/2 cup cherry tomatoes, halved
- Salt and pepper to taste
- Cooking spray or oil for greasing the skillet

Preparation Method:
1. Preheat your oven to 350°F (175°C).
2. Whisk the eggs and milk together thoroughly in a mixing bowl. To taste, add salt and pepper for seasoning.
3. Heat an oven-safe skillet over medium heat and lightly grease it with cooking spray or oil.
4. Add spinach leaves to the skillet and cook until wilted, about 2-3 minutes.
5. Pour the egg mixture into the skillet over the spinach.
6. Sprinkle crumbled feta cheese evenly over the eggs.
7. Arrange cherry tomato halves on top of the frittata.
8. Cook on the stovetop for 3-4 minutes until the edges start to set.

9. Transfer the skillet to the preheated oven and bake for 12-15 minutes, or until the frittata is set and golden brown on top.
10. Take out of the oven and allow it to cool down a little before slicing.
11. Serve warm or at room temperature.
12. Enjoy your flavorful spinach and feta frittata with cherry tomatoes as a satisfying breakfast or brunch option.

Overnight Oats with Almond Milk, Chia Seeds, and Mixed Berries

Ingredients:
- 1/2 cup rolled oats
- 1 tablespoon chia seeds
- 1/2 cup almond milk (or any milk of your choice)
- Half a cup of mixed berries, including raspberries, blueberries, and strawberries.
- One tablespoon (optional) of maple syrup or honey.
- Optional toppings: sliced almonds, shredded coconut, additional berries

Preparation Method:
1. In a mason jar or airtight container, combine the rolled oats, chia seeds, almond milk, and honey or maple syrup (if using). Stir well to combine.
2. Add the mixed berries to the mixture and gently stir to distribute them evenly.
3. Cover the jar or container with a lid and refrigerate overnight, or for at least 4 hours, to allow

the oats and chia seeds to soften and absorb the liquid.

4. In the morning, give the overnight oats a good stir.

5. If desired, top with sliced almonds, shredded coconut, and additional berries before serving.

6. Enjoy your delicious and convenient overnight oats with almond milk, chia seeds, and mixed berries.

Egg White and Vegetable Breakfast Burrito with Salsa Verde

Ingredients:
- 3 large egg whites
- 1/4 cup of bell peppers, chopped, any color.
- 1/4 cup diced onions
- 1/4 cup diced tomatoes
- 1/4 cup chopped spinach leaves
- Salt and pepper to taste
- 1 whole wheat tortilla
- 2 tablespoons salsa verde

Preparation Method:

1. In a non-stick skillet, sauté the diced bell peppers and onions over medium heat until softened, about 3-4 minutes.

2. Add the diced tomatoes and chopped spinach to the skillet and cook for an additional 1-2 minutes, until the spinach wilts.

3. To taste, add salt and pepper to the vegetables.

4. Pour the egg whites over the cooked vegetables in the skillet.

5. Cook, stirring occasionally, until the egg whites are set and cooked through, about 2-3 minutes.
6. Warm the whole wheat tortilla in the microwave or on a skillet until pliable.
7. Spoon the cooked egg white and vegetable mixture onto the center of the tortilla.
8. Top with salsa verde.
9. Fold in the sides of the tortilla and roll it up tightly to form a burrito.
10. Serve immediately and enjoy your flavorful egg white and vegetable breakfast burrito with salsa verse.

Whole Wheat Bagel with Low-Fat Cream Cheese and Sliced Cucumbers

Ingredients:
- One bagel made of whole wheat, cut and toasted.
- 2 tablespoons low-fat cream cheese
- 1/2 cucumber, thinly sliced

Preparation Method:
1. Toast the sliced whole wheat bagel until golden brown and crispy.
2. Spread low-fat cream cheese evenly on each bagel half.
3. Arrange thinly sliced cucumber on top of the cream cheese.
4. Serve immediately and enjoy your satisfying whole wheat bagel with low-fat cream cheese and sliced cucumbers.

Buckwheat Crepes Filled with Greek Yogurt and Fresh Fruit
Ingredients:
For the Buckwheat Crepes:
- 1 cup buckwheat flour
- 2 large eggs
- 1 cup milk (almond milk, soy milk, or regular milk)
- 1/4 teaspoon salt
- Greasing the skillet with butter or cooking spray.

For the Filling:
- One cup of plain or flavored Greek yogurt.
- Assorted fresh fruits (such as strawberries, blueberries, bananas, etc.), sliced

Preparation Method:
For the Buckwheat Crepes:
1. In a mixing bowl, whisk together the buckwheat flour, eggs, milk, and salt until smooth.
2. Heat a non-stick skillet over medium heat and lightly grease it with cooking spray or butter.
3. Pour about 1/4 cup of the batter onto the skillet, swirling to spread it thinly.
4. Cook for one to two minutes, or until the bottom is golden brown and the edges begin to lift.
5. Flip the crepe and cook for an additional 1-2 minutes until cooked through.
6. Repeat with the remaining batter, stacking the cooked crepes on a plate.

For the Filling:
1. Spread Greek yogurt on each crepe.

2. Add sliced fresh fruits on one half of each crepe.

3. Fold the crepes in half and then into quarters.

4. Serve immediately and enjoy your delicious buckwheat crepes filled with Greek yogurt and fresh fruit.

Breakfast Quinoa Bowl with Sliced Peaches, Almonds, and Honey

Ingredients:

- 1 cup cooked quinoa
- 1 ripe peach, sliced
- 2 tablespoons sliced almonds
- Honey for drizzling

Preparation Method:

1. In a serving bowl, spoon the cooked quinoa.

2. Arrange the sliced peaches and sliced almonds on top of the quinoa.

3. Drizzle with honey for sweetness.

4. Serve immediately and enjoy your nutritious breakfast quinoa bowl with sliced peaches, almonds, and honey.

Baked Sweet Potato Topped with Greek Yogurt and Cinnamon

Ingredients:

- 1 medium sweet potato
- 1/2 cup Greek yogurt (plain or flavored)
- Ground cinnamon for sprinkling

Preparation Method:

1. Preheat your oven to 400°F (200°C).

2. Wash the sweet potato and pat dry.

3. Pierce the sweet potato several times with a fork.

4. Place the sweet potato on a baking sheet and bake for 45-60 minutes, or until tender.

5. Remove the sweet potato from the oven and let it cool slightly.

6. Slice open the sweet potato lengthwise and fluff the flesh with a fork.

7. Top with Greek yogurt and sprinkle with ground cinnamon.

8. Serve immediately and enjoy your baked sweet potato topped with Greek yogurt and cinnamon as a nutritious breakfast or snack option.

Low-Fat Cheese and Tomato Sandwich on Whole Grain Bread

Ingredients:
- 2 slices whole grain bread
- 2 slices low-fat cheese
- 1 ripe tomato, thinly sliced
- Lettuce leaves
- Mustard or mayonnaise (optional)
- Salt and pepper to taste

Preparation Method:
1. Place the slices of whole grain bread on a clean surface.

2. Layer one slice of bread with lettuce leaves, followed by tomato slices.

3. Season the tomatoes with salt and pepper to taste.

4. Add the slices of low-fat cheese on top of the tomatoes.

5. If desired, spread mustard or mayonnaise on the other slice of bread.

6. Place the second slice of bread over the cheese to form a sandwich.

7. Cut the sandwich in half if desired.

8. Serve immediately and enjoy your delicious low-fat cheese and tomato sandwich on whole grain bread.

Spinach and Mushroom Crustless Quiche

Ingredients:
- 1 tablespoon olive oil
- 1 cup sliced mushrooms
- 2 cups fresh spinach leaves
- 6 large eggs
- Half a cup of milk (normal, soy, or almond).
- Salt and pepper to taste
- 1/2 cup shredded low-fat cheese (optional)

Preparation Method:
1. Preheat your oven to 375°F (190°C). Lightly grease a pie dish or quiche pan with cooking spray or oil.

2. Heat olive oil in a skillet over medium heat.

3. Add sliced mushrooms to the skillet and cook until they release their moisture and become tender, about 5 minutes.

4. Add fresh spinach leaves to the skillet and cook until wilted, about 2-3 minutes.

5. In a mixing bowl, whisk together eggs and milk until well combined. To taste, add salt and pepper for seasoning.

6. Spread the cooked mushrooms and spinach evenly in the greased pie dish or quiche pan.
7. Pour the egg mixture over the mushrooms and spinach.
8. If desired, sprinkle shredded low-fat cheese on top of the egg mixture.
9. Bake in the preheated oven for 25-30 minutes, or until the quiche is set and the top is golden brown.
10. Remove from the oven and let it cool slightly before slicing.
11. Serve warm or at room temperature.
12. Enjoy your delicious spinach and mushroom crustless quiche as a satisfying breakfast or brunch option.

Breakfast Tacos with Scrambled Eggs, Black Beans, and Avocado
Ingredients:
- 4 small whole wheat tortillas
- 4 large eggs, scrambled
- 1 cup cooked black beans
- 1 ripe avocado, sliced
- Salsa or hot sauce (optional)
- Fresh cilantro leaves (optional)
- Lime wedges (optional)
- Salt and pepper to taste

Preparation Method:
1. Warm the whole wheat tortillas in a skillet or microwave until heated through.

2. In a skillet, scramble the eggs until cooked to your desired doneness. To taste, add salt and pepper for seasoning.
3. Warm the black beans in a small saucepan over medium heat.
4. Assemble the tacos by placing scrambled eggs, black beans, and avocado slices on each tortilla.
5. If desired, top with salsa or hot sauce, fresh cilantro leaves, and a squeeze of lime juice.
6. Serve immediately and enjoy your flavorful breakfast tacos with scrambled eggs, black beans, and avocado.

Coconut Milk Chia Seed Pudding with Sliced Mango and Pistachios
Ingredients:
- 1/4 cup chia seeds
- 1 cup coconut milk (canned or carton)
- 1 ripe mango, sliced
- 2 tablespoons pistachios, chopped
- For sweetness, optional: honey or maple syrup.

Preparation Method:
1. In a mixing bowl, combine the chia seeds and coconut milk.
2. If desired, sweeten with honey or maple syrup and thoroughly combine.
3. Cover the bowl and refrigerate for at least 4 hours or overnight, allowing the chia seeds to absorb the coconut milk and thicken.
4. Once the chia pudding is set, give it a good stir.

5. Spoon the chia seed pudding into serving bowls or glasses.
6. Top with sliced mango and chopped pistachios.
7. Serve chilled and enjoy your delightful coconut milk chia seed pudding with sliced mango and pistachios.

Whole Grain Toast with Ricotta Cheese and Sliced Strawberries

Ingredients:
- 2 slices whole grain bread, toasted
- 1/2 cup ricotta cheese
- 1 cup sliced strawberries
- Honey or balsamic glaze for drizzling is optional.

Preparation Method:
1. Spread ricotta cheese evenly on each slice of toasted whole grain bread.
2. Arrange sliced strawberries on top of the ricotta cheese.
3. If desired, drizzle with honey or balsamic glaze for added flavor.
4. Serve immediately and enjoy your nutritious whole grain toast with ricotta cheese and sliced strawberries.

Egg White and Vegetable Breakfast Sandwich on a Whole Wheat English Muffin

Ingredients:
- 2 whole wheat English muffins, split and toasted
- 4 large egg whites
- 1/4 cup of bell peppers, chopped, any color.

- 1/4 cup diced onions
- 1/4 cup diced tomatoes
- 1/4 cup chopped spinach leaves
- Salt and pepper to taste

Preparation Method:
1. In a non-stick skillet, sauté the diced bell peppers and onions over medium heat until softened, about 3-4 minutes.
2. Add the diced tomatoes and chopped spinach to the skillet and cook for an additional 1-2 minutes, until the spinach wilts.
3. To taste, add salt and pepper to the vegetables.
4. In another skillet, scramble the egg whites until cooked through. To taste, add salt and pepper for seasoning.
5. To assemble the sandwich, place a portion of scrambled egg whites on the bottom half of each toasted English muffin.
6. Top with sautéed vegetables.
7. Cover with the top half of the English muffin.
8. Serve immediately and enjoy your delicious egg white and vegetable breakfast sandwich on a whole wheat English muffin.

Breakfast Wrap with Turkey Slices, Lettuce, and Hummus
Ingredients:
- 1 large whole wheat tortilla
- 3-4 slices of turkey breast
- 1-2 large lettuce leaves
- 2 tablespoons hummus

Preparation Method:
1. Lay the whole wheat tortilla flat on a clean surface.
2. Spread hummus evenly over the center of the tortilla.
3. Place the turkey slices on top of the hummus.
4. Lay the lettuce leaves over the turkey slices.
5. Fold in the sides of the tortilla and then roll it up tightly to form a wrap.
6. Serve immediately and enjoy your nutritious breakfast wrap with turkey slices, lettuce, and hummus.

Low-Fat Yogurt with Sliced Figs and Crushed Pistachios

Ingredients:
- 1 cup low-fat yogurt (plain or flavored)
- 2-3 fresh figs, sliced
- 2 tablespoons crushed pistachios

Preparation Method:
1. Spoon the low-fat yogurt into a serving bowl.
2. Arrange the sliced figs on top of the yogurt.
3. Sprinkle crushed pistachios over the figs and yogurt.
4. Serve immediately and enjoy your delightful low-fat yogurt with sliced figs and crushed pistachios.

Baked Apple Oatmeal Topped with Greek Yogurt and Maple Syrup
Ingredients:
- 1 cup rolled oats
- 1 apple, peeled, cored, and diced
- 1 teaspoon ground cinnamon
- 1/4 teaspoon ground nutmeg
- 2 cups milk (almond milk, soy milk, or regular milk)
- 1/4 cup maple syrup
- 1/2 cup Greek yogurt (plain or flavored)

Preparation Method:
1. Preheat your oven to 375°F (190°C). Grease a baking dish with cooking spray or butter.
2. In a mixing bowl, combine the rolled oats, diced apple, ground cinnamon, and ground nutmeg.
3. Spread the oat mixture evenly in the prepared baking dish.
4. In another bowl, whisk together the milk and maple syrup until well combined.
5. Pour the milk mixture over the oat mixture in the baking dish.
6. Bake in the preheated oven for 35-40 minutes, or until the oatmeal is cooked through and the top is golden brown.
7. Take out of the oven and allow to cool down a little.
8. Serve the baked apple oatmeal warm, topped with Greek yogurt and an extra drizzle of maple syrup if desired.

9. Enjoy your comforting baked apple oatmeal topped with Greek yogurt and maple syrup for a satisfying breakfast option

Breakfast Pizza with Whole Wheat Crust, Scrambled Eggs, and Veggies
Ingredients:
For the Whole Wheat Crust:
- 1 cup whole wheat flour
- 1 teaspoon baking powder
- 1/4 teaspoon salt
- 1/2 cup plain Greek yogurt

For the Toppings:
- 4 large eggs, scrambled
- Assorted chopped vegetables (bell peppers, onions, mushrooms, spinach, etc.)
- 1/2 cup shredded low-fat cheese
- Salt and pepper to taste

Preparation Method:
For the Whole Wheat Crust:
1. Preheat your oven to 425°F (220°C).
2. In a mixing bowl, combine the whole wheat flour, baking powder, and salt.
3. Stir in the Greek yogurt until a dough forms.
4. Place the dough onto a surface dusted with flour and knead it until it becomes smooth.
5. Roll out the dough into a circle or rectangle, depending on your preference.
6. Transfer the crust to a baking sheet lined with parchment paper.

For the Pizza:

1. Spread the scrambled eggs evenly over the prepared whole wheat crust.

2. Top with assorted chopped vegetables and shredded low-fat cheese.

3. To taste, add salt and pepper for seasoning.

4. Bake in the preheated oven for 15-20 minutes, or until the crust is golden brown and the toppings are heated through.

5. Remove from the oven and let cool slightly before slicing.

6. Serve hot and enjoy your delicious breakfast pizza with whole wheat crust, scrambled eggs, and veggies.

Whole Grain Cereal with Skim Milk and Fresh Berries

Ingredients:

- 1 cup whole grain cereal (such as oats, bran flakes, or whole wheat flakes)
- 1 cup skim milk
- Half a cup of fresh berries, like raspberries, blueberries, and strawberries

Preparation Method:

1. Place the whole grain cereal in a bowl.
2. Pour skim milk over the cereal.
3. Top with fresh berries.

4. Serve immediately and enjoy your nutritious whole grain cereal with skim milk and fresh berries.

Quinoa Breakfast Bowl with Poached Egg, Avocado, and Salsa

Ingredients:
- 1/2 cup cooked quinoa
- 1 poached egg
- 1/4 avocado, sliced
- 2 tablespoons salsa
- Salt and pepper to taste

Preparation Method:
1. Spoon the cooked quinoa into a serving bowl.
2. Top with a poached egg and sliced avocado.
3. Spoon salsa over the quinoa, egg, and avocado.
4. To taste, add salt and pepper for seasoning.
5. Serve immediately and enjoy your flavorful quinoa breakfast bowl with poached egg, avocado, and salsa.

Egg White and Turkey Sausage Muffins with Spinach and Bell Peppers

Ingredients:
- 6 egg whites
- 4 turkey sausage patties, cooked and crumbled
- 1 cup spinach, chopped
- 1/2 cup bell peppers, diced
- Salt and pepper to taste
- Cooking spray

Preparation Method:
1. Preheat your oven to 350°F (175°C). Put cooking spray to a muffin tin and grease it.
2. In a mixing bowl, whisk together the egg whites, cooked and crumbled turkey sausage, chopped spinach, diced bell peppers, salt, and pepper.
3. Pour the egg mixture evenly into the prepared muffin tin, filling each cup about 3/4 full.
4. Bake in the preheated oven for 20-25 minutes, or until the muffins are set and lightly golden on top.
5. Take out of the oven and allow it to cool down a little before serving.
6. Enjoy your tasty egg white and turkey sausage muffins with spinach and bell peppers as a nutritious breakfast option.

Rice Cake with Almond Butter and Sliced Apples
Ingredients:
- 1 rice cake
- 1 tablespoon almond butter
- 1/2 apple, thinly sliced

Preparation Method:
1. Spread almond butter evenly over the rice cake.
2. Arrange thinly sliced apples on top of the almond butter.
3. Serve immediately and enjoy your simple yet delicious rice cake with almond butter and sliced apples.

Low-Fat Cottage Cheese with Pear Slices and Cinnamon

Ingredients:
- 1/2 cup low-fat cottage cheese
- 1 ripe pear, sliced
- Ground cinnamon for sprinkling

Preparation Method:
1. Spoon the low-fat cottage cheese into a serving bowl.
2. Arrange the sliced pears on top of the cottage cheese.
3. Sprinkle ground cinnamon over the cottage cheese and pears.
4. Serve immediately and enjoy your nutritious low-fat cottage cheese with pear slices and cinnamon.

Breakfast Burrito Bowl with Brown Rice, Black Beans, and Salsa

Ingredients:
- 1 cup cooked brown rice
- 1/2 cup washed and drained canned black beans.
- 1/4 cup salsa
- Optional toppings: sliced avocado, chopped cilantro, Greek yogurt, lime wedges

Preparation Method:
1. In a serving bowl, layer cooked brown rice and black beans.
2. Top with salsa and any optional toppings of your choice.

3. Serve immediately and enjoy your flavorful breakfast burrito bowl with brown rice, black beans, and salsa.

Breakfast Sandwich with Spinach and Tomato on Whole Grain Bread
Ingredients:
- 2 slices whole grain bread, toasted
- 1/2 cup fresh spinach leaves
- 1 tomato, sliced
- 2 eggs, scrambled
- Salt and pepper to taste

Preparation Method:
1. On one slice of toasted whole grain bread, layer fresh spinach leaves and sliced tomato.
2. Top with scrambled eggs seasoned with salt and pepper.
3. Place the second slice of toasted bread on top to form a sandwich.
4. Serve immediately and enjoy your nutritious spinach and tomato breakfast sandwich on whole grain bread.

Buckwheat Granola with Low-Fat Yogurt and Mixed Fruit
Ingredients:
For the Buckwheat Granola:
- 1 cup buckwheat groats
- 1/4 cup honey or maple syrup
- 1 tablespoon coconut oil, melted
- 1 teaspoon ground cinnamon

- 1/2 cup chopped nuts or seeds (such as almonds, walnuts, pumpkin seeds)
- 1/4 cup dried fruit (such as raisins, cranberries, chopped apricots)

For Serving:
- 1 cup low-fat yogurt (plain or flavored)
- 1 cup mixed fresh fruit (such as berries, sliced bananas, diced apples)

Preparation Method:
1. Preheat your oven to 325°F (160°C). Line a baking sheet with parchment paper.
2. In a mixing bowl, combine the buckwheat groats, honey or maple syrup, melted coconut oil, and ground cinnamon. Stir until well combined.
3. Spread the mixture evenly on the prepared baking sheet.
4. Bake in the preheated oven for 20-25 minutes, stirring occasionally, until the granola is golden brown and crisp.
5. Take out of the oven and allow it cool fully.
6. Once cooled, stir in the chopped nuts or seeds and dried fruit.
7. To serve, divide the low-fat yogurt into serving bowls.
8. Top with the buckwheat granola and mixed fresh fruit.
9. Serve immediately and enjoy your delicious buckwheat granola with low-fat yogurt and mixed fruit.

Egg White and Vegetable Frittata Muffins with Salsa

Ingredients:
- 8 large egg whites
- 1/2 cup diced bell peppers (any color)
- 1/2 cup diced onions
- 1/2 cup diced tomatoes
- 1/2 cup chopped spinach leaves
- Salt and pepper to taste
- Cooking spray
- Salsa for serving

Preparation Method:
1. Preheat your oven to 350°F (175°C). Put cooking spray to a muffin tin and grease it.
2. In a mixing bowl, whisk together the egg whites until frothy.
3. Stir in the diced bell peppers, onions, tomatoes, and chopped spinach.
4. To taste, add salt and pepper for seasoning.
5. Pour the egg mixture evenly into the prepared muffin tin, filling each cup about 3/4 full.
6. Bake in the preheated oven for 20-25 minutes, or until the frittata muffins are set and lightly golden on top.
7. Remove from the oven and let cool slightly before removing from the muffin tin.
8. Serve the frittata muffins warm or at room temperature with salsa on the side.
9. Enjoy your tasty egg white and vegetable frittata muffins with salsa as a nutritious breakfast or snack option!

Cottage Cheese and Fruit Salad with Honey and Mint
Ingredients:
- 1 cup low-fat cottage cheese
- 1 cup mixed fresh fruit (such as berries, grapes, melon, kiwi)
- 1 tablespoon honey
- Fresh mint leaves for garnish

Preparation Method:
1. In a serving bowl, spoon the low-fat cottage cheese.
2. Add the mixed fresh fruit to the bowl.
3. Drizzle honey over the cottage cheese and fruit.
4. Gently toss to coat the fruit in honey.
5. Garnish with fresh mint leaves.
6. Serve immediately and enjoy your refreshing cottage cheese and fruit salad with honey and mint.

Smoothies

Here are smoothie ideas suitable for individuals without a gallbladder:

1. Banana Berry Blast
   Greek yogurt, spinach, almond milk, banana, and mixed berries are among the ingredients.

2. Tropical Paradise
   Ingredients: Pineapple, mango, banana, coconut water, spinach.

3. Green Goddess

Ingredients: Spinach, kale, cucumber, apple, lemon juice, coconut water.

4. Peanut Butter Power

Ingredients: Banana, peanut butter, oats, almond milk, Greek yogurt.

5. Mango Tango

Ingredients: Mango, orange, banana, Greek yogurt, almond milk.

6. Berry Beet Boost

Ingredients: Mixed berries, cooked beets, spinach, almond milk, honey.

7. Peachy Keen

Ingredients: Peach, banana, spinach, almond milk, Greek yogurt.

8. Chocolate Avocado Dream

Ingredients: Avocado, cocoa powder, banana, almond milk, Greek yogurt.

9. Blueberry Bliss

Ingredients: Blueberries, banana, spinach, almond milk, Greek yogurt.

10. Creamy Coconut Pineapple

Ingredients: Pineapple, coconut milk, banana, spinach, Greek yogurt.

11. Citrus Sunshine
   Ingredients: Orange, mango, banana, Greek yogurt, almond milk.

12. Strawberry Spinach Delight
   Ingredients: Strawberries, spinach, banana, almond milk, Greek yogurt.

13. Cherry Almond Bliss
   Ingredients: Cherries, almond milk, banana, spinach, Greek yogurt.

14. Apple Cinnamon Swirl
   Ingredients: Apple, banana, cinnamon, oats, almond milk, Greek yogurt.

15. Raspberry Lemonade Smoothie
   Ingredients: Raspberries, lemon juice, banana, almond milk, Greek yogurt.

16. Kiwi Kale Kickstart
   Ingredients: Kiwi, kale, banana, almond milk, Greek yogurt.

17. Orange Creamsicle
   Ingredients: Orange, banana, vanilla extract, almond milk, Greek yogurt.

18. Pineapple Coconut Green Smoothie
   Ingredients: Pineapple, coconut water, spinach, banana, Greek yogurt.

19. Pomegranate Power Punch
     Ingredients: Pomegranate seeds, banana, almond milk, spinach, Greek yogurt.

20. Banana Bread Smoothie
    Ingredients: Banana, oats, cinnamon, almond milk, Greek yogurt.

21. Vanilla Blueberry Smoothie
    Ingredients: Blueberries, banana, vanilla extract, almond milk, Greek yogurt.

22. Watermelon Mint Cooler
     - Ingredients: Watermelon, mint leaves, cucumber, lime juice, Greek yogurt.

23. Raspberry Mango Tango
     - Ingredients: Raspberries, mango, banana, almond milk, Greek yogurt.

24. Chocolate Cherry Bomb
     - Ingredients: Cherries, cocoa powder, banana, almond milk, Greek yogurt.

25. Green Apple Ginger Zing
     - Ingredients: Green apple, ginger, spinach, banana, almond milk, Greek yogurt.

26. Strawberry Banana Protein Smoothie
     Ingredients: Strawberries, banana, protein powder, almond milk, Greek yogurt.

27. Blueberry Kale Crush
    Ingredients: Blueberries, kale, banana, almond milk, Greek yogurt.

28. Mango Pineapple Paradise
    Ingredients: Mango, pineapple, banana, almond milk, Greek yogurt.

29. Peach Raspberry Delight
    Ingredients: Peach, raspberries, banana, almond milk, Greek yogurt.

30. Chocolate Peanut Butter Protein Smoothie
    Ingredients: Cocoa powder, peanut butter, banana, almond milk, Greek yogurt.

31. Tropical Green Smoothie
    Ingredients: Pineapple, mango, banana, spinach, coconut water.

32. Blueberry Avocado Delight
    Ingredients: Blueberries, avocado, banana, almond milk, Greek yogurt.

33. Strawberry Kiwi Cooler
    Ingredients: Strawberries, kiwi, banana, almond milk, Greek yogurt.

34. Raspberry Coconut Dream
    Ingredients: Raspberries, coconut milk, banana, almond milk, Greek yogurt.

35. Almond Joy Smoothie
   Ingredients: Almond milk, cocoa powder, almond butter, banana, coconut flakes.

36. Mango Mint Madness
   Ingredients: Mango, mint leaves, banana, coconut water, Greek yogurt.

37. Green Grape Glory
   Ingredients: Green grapes, banana, spinach, almond milk, Greek yogurt.

38. Cherry Chocolate Chip Smoothie
   Ingredients: Cherries, cocoa powder, banana, almond milk, Greek yogurt.

39. Banana Coconut Chia Smoothie
   Ingredients: Banana, coconut milk, chia seeds, almond milk, Greek yogurt.

40. Pineapple Orange Sunshine Smoothie
   Ingredients: Pineapple, orange, banana, almond milk, Greek yogurt.

41. Raspberry Lemon Smoothie
   Ingredients: Raspberries, lemon juice, banana, almond milk, Greek yogurt.

42. Blueberry Spinach Burst
   Ingredients: Blueberries, spinach, banana, almond milk, Greek yogurt.

43. Mango Peach Paradise
      Ingredients: Mango, peach, banana, almond milk, Greek yogurt.

44. Apple Cinnamon Oatmeal Smoothie
      Ingredients: Apple, oats, cinnamon, banana, almond milk, Greek yogurt.

45. Strawberry Banana Coconut Smoothie
   Ingredients: Strawberries, banana, coconut milk, almond milk, Greek yogurt.

46. Pineapple Strawberry Splash
      Ingredients: Pineapple, strawberries, banana, almond milk, Greek yogurt.

47. Mango Lime Mojito Smoothie
      Ingredients: Mango, lime juice, mint leaves, banana, almond milk, Greek yogurt.

48. Blackberry Banana Blast
   Ingredients: Blackberries, banana, almond milk, spinach, Greek yogurt.

49. Chocolate Raspberry Dream
   Ingredients: Raspberries, cocoa powder, banana, almond milk, Greek yogurt.

50. Spinach Avocado Smoothie
      Ingredients: Spinach, avocado, banana, almond milk, Greek yogurt.

51. Mango Pineapple Kale Smoothie
    Ingredients: Mango, pineapple, kale, banana, almond milk, Greek yogurt.

52. Blueberry Pomegranate Smoothie
    Ingredients: Blueberries, pomegranate seeds, banana, almond milk, Greek yogurt.

53. Chocolate Banana Nut Smoothie
    Ingredients: Cocoa powder, banana, almond milk, peanut butter, Greek yogurt.

54. Strawberry Peach Smoothie
    Ingredients: Strawberries, peach, banana, almond milk, Greek yogurt.

55. Kiwi Pineapple Smoothie
    Ingredients: Kiwi, pineapple, banana, spinach, almond milk, Greek yogurt.

Basic Smoothie Recipe
Ingredients:
- 1 cup frozen fruits (such as berries, mango, pineapple)
- 1 ripe banana, fresh or frozen
- 1 cup leafy greens (such as spinach, kale)
- 1/2 cup Greek yogurt (plain or flavored)
- 1-1.5 cups liquid (water, coconut water, almond milk, or soy milk)
- Optional add-ins: chia seeds, flaxseeds, protein powder, honey, or maple syrup for sweetness

Preparation Method:
1. Add the frozen fruits, banana, leafy greens, and Greek yogurt to a blender.
2. Pour in the liquid of your choice.
3. Optionally, add any desired add-ins for extra nutrition or sweetness.
4. Blend until smooth and creamy, adding more liquid if necessary to reach your desired consistency.
5. Taste the smoothie and adjust sweetness or thickness by adding more sweeteners or liquid, if needed.
6. Once blended to your liking, pour the smoothie into glasses and serve immediately.
7. Enjoy your nutritious and delicious smoothie as a refreshing and healthy snack or meal replacement.
Note: Follow the method for any other smoothie of your choice

Oatmeal Variations

Here are various oatmeal variations suitable for individuals without a gallbladder:

Classic Oatmeal Recipe
Ingredients:
- 1/2 cup rolled oats (old-fashioned oats)
- 1 cup water or milk (almond milk, soy milk, or regular milk)
- Pinch of salt (optional)
- Toppings of your choice: sliced fruits, nuts, seeds, honey, cinnamon, etc.

Preparation Method:
1. In a small saucepan, bring the water or milk to a gentle boil over medium heat.
2. Stir in the rolled oats and salt (if using).
3. Reduce the heat to low and simmer the oats, stirring occasionally, for about 5-7 minutes or until the oats are tender and the mixture thickens to your desired consistency.
4. Once the oats are cooked, remove the saucepan from the heat.
5. Transfer the cooked oatmeal to a serving bowl.
6. Add your favorite toppings such as sliced fruits, nuts, seeds, honey, or cinnamon.
7. Stir well to combine the toppings with the oatmeal.
8. Let the oatmeal cool slightly before serving.
9. Enjoy your classic oatmeal as a nutritious and comforting breakfast option!

Note: For a creamier texture, you can use milk instead of water. Additionally, you can adjust the consistency of the oatmeal by adding more or less liquid according to your preference.

Banana Oatmeal
Ingredients:
- 1/2 cup rolled oats
- 1 cup water or milk (almond milk, soy milk, or regular milk)
- 1 ripe banana, mashed
- Pinch of salt (optional)

- Toppings: Sliced bananas, honey or maple syrup, chopped nuts (optional)

Preparation Method:
1. In a small saucepan, bring the water or milk to a gentle boil over medium heat.
2. Stir in the rolled oats and salt (if using).
3. Reduce the heat to low and simmer, stirring occasionally, for about 5-7 minutes or until the oats are tender and the mixture thickens.
4. Once the oats are cooked, remove the saucepan from the heat.
5. Stir in the mashed banana until well combined.
6. Transfer the banana oatmeal to a serving bowl.
7. Top with sliced bananas, a drizzle of honey or maple syrup, and chopped nuts if desired.
8. Serve warm and enjoy your delicious banana oatmeal.

Berry Blast Oatmeal

Ingredients:
- 1/2 cup rolled oats
- 1 cup water or milk (almond milk, soy milk, or regular milk)
- 1/2 cup mixed berries (such as strawberries, blueberries, raspberries)
- Pinch of salt (optional)
- Toppings: Fresh berries, honey or maple syrup, sliced almonds (optional)

Preparation Method:
1. Follow the same preparation method as for basic oatmeal (see previous recipe).

2. When the oatmeal is almost done cooking, stir in the mixed berries.
3. Continue to cook for an additional 1-2 minutes until the berries soften slightly.
4. Remove from heat and transfer the berry oatmeal to a serving bowl.
5. Top with fresh berries, a drizzle of honey or maple syrup, and sliced almonds if desired.
6. Serve warm and enjoy your flavorful berry blast oatmeal.

Apple Cinnamon Oatmeal

Ingredients:
- 1/2 cup rolled oats
- 1 cup water or milk (almond milk, soy milk, or regular milk)
- 1/2 apple, peeled, cored, and diced
- Pinch of ground cinnamon
- Pinch of salt (optional)
- Toppings: Sliced apples, a sprinkle of cinnamon, chopped walnuts (optional)

Preparation Method:
1. Follow the same preparation method as for basic oatmeal (see previous recipe).
2. When the oatmeal is almost done cooking, stir in the diced apple and ground cinnamon.
3. Continue to cook for an additional 1-2 minutes until the apples are tender.
4. Remove from heat and transfer the apple cinnamon oatmeal to a serving bowl.

5. Top with sliced apples, a sprinkle of cinnamon, and chopped walnuts if desired.
6. Serve warm and enjoy your comforting apple cinnamon oatmeal.

Peanut Butter Banana Oatmeal
Ingredients:
- 1/2 cup rolled oats
- 1 cup water or milk (almond milk, soy milk, or regular milk)
- 1 ripe banana, mashed
- 1-2 tablespoons peanut butter
- Pinch of salt (optional)
- Toppings: Sliced bananas, a drizzle of honey or maple syrup, chopped peanuts (optional)

Preparation Method:
1. Follow the same preparation method as for basic oatmeal (see previous recipe).
2. When the oatmeal is almost done cooking, stir in the mashed banana and peanut butter.
3. Continue to cook for an additional 1-2 minutes until the mixture is creamy and well combined.
4. Remove from heat and transfer the peanut butter banana oatmeal to a serving bowl.
5. Top with sliced bananas, a drizzle of honey or maple syrup, and chopped peanuts if desired.
6. Serve warm and enjoy your delicious peanut butter banana oatmeal.

Coconut Almond Oatmeal

Ingredients:
- 1/2 cup rolled oats
- 1 cup water or milk (almond milk, soy milk, or regular milk)
- 2 tablespoons shredded coconut
- 2 tablespoons chopped almonds
- Pinch of salt (optional)
- Toppings: Toasted coconut flakes, sliced almonds, drizzle of honey (optional)

Preparation Method:
1. In a small saucepan, bring the water or milk to a gentle boil over medium heat.
2. Stir in the rolled oats, shredded coconut, chopped almonds, and salt (if using).
3. Reduce the heat to low and simmer, stirring occasionally, for about 5-7 minutes or until the oats are tender and the mixture thickens.
4. Once the oats are cooked, remove the saucepan from the heat.
5. Transfer the coconut almond oatmeal to a serving bowl.
6. Top with toasted coconut flakes, sliced almonds, and a drizzle of honey if desired.
7. Serve warm and enjoy your comforting coconut almond oatmeal.

Chocolate Banana Oatmeal

Ingredients:
- 1/2 cup rolled oats

- 1 cup water or milk (almond milk, soy milk, or regular milk)
- 1 ripe banana, mashed
- 1 tablespoon cocoa powder
- Pinch of salt (optional)
- Toppings: Sliced bananas, chocolate chips, chopped nuts (optional)

Preparation Method:
1. Follow the same preparation method as for basic oatmeal (see previous recipe).
2. When the oatmeal is almost done cooking, stir in the mashed banana and cocoa powder.
3. Continue to cook for an additional 1-2 minutes until the mixture is creamy and well combined.
4. Remove from heat and transfer the chocolate banana oatmeal to a serving bowl.
5. Top with sliced bananas, chocolate chips, and chopped nuts if desired.
6. Serve warm and enjoy your indulgent chocolate banana oatmeal.

Pumpkin Spice Oatmeal
Ingredients:
- 1/2 cup rolled oats
- 1 cup water or milk (almond milk, soy milk, or regular milk)
- 1/4 cup canned pumpkin puree
- 1/2 teaspoon pumpkin pie spice
- Pinch of salt (optional)
- Toppings: Maple syrup, chopped pecans, dash of cinnamon (optional)

Preparation Method:
1. Follow the same preparation method as for basic oatmeal (see previous recipe).
2. When the oatmeal is almost done cooking, stir in the pumpkin puree and pumpkin pie spice.
3. Continue to cook for an additional 1-2 minutes until the mixture is heated through and well combined.
4. Remove from heat and transfer the pumpkin spice oatmeal to a serving bowl.
5. Top with maple syrup, chopped pecans, and a dash of cinnamon if desired.
6. Serve warm and enjoy your cozy pumpkin spice oatmeal.

Blueberry Lemon Oatmeal
Ingredients:
- 1/2 cup rolled oats
- 1 cup water or milk (almond milk, soy milk, or regular milk)
- 1/2 cup fresh or frozen blueberries
- Zest of 1 lemon
- Pinch of salt (optional)
- Toppings: Fresh blueberries, lemon slices, drizzle of honey (optional)

Preparation Method:
1. Follow the same preparation method as for basic oatmeal (see previous recipe).
2. When the oatmeal is almost done cooking, stir in the blueberries and lemon zest.

3. Continue to cook for an additional 1-2 minutes until the blueberries soften slightly.
4. Remove from heat and transfer the blueberry lemon oatmeal to a serving bowl.
5. Top with fresh blueberries, lemon slices, and a drizzle of honey if desired.
6. Serve warm and enjoy your refreshing blueberry lemon oatmeal.

Peach Cobbler Oatmeal
Ingredients:
- 1/2 cup rolled oats
- 1 cup water or milk (almond milk, soy milk, or regular milk)
- One mature peach, chopped, pitted, and peeled
- 1/4 teaspoon ground cinnamon
- Pinch of salt (optional)
- Toppings: Sliced peaches, granola, sprinkle of cinnamon (optional)

Preparation Method:
1. Follow the same preparation method as for basic oatmeal (see previous recipe).
2. When the oatmeal is almost done cooking, stir in the diced peach and ground cinnamon.
3. Continue to cook for an additional 1-2 minutes until the peach is tender.
4. Remove from heat and transfer the peach cobbler oatmeal to a serving bowl.
5. Top with sliced peaches, granola, and a sprinkle of cinnamon if desired.

6. Serve warm and enjoy your delightful peach cobbler oatmeal.

Cherry Almond Oatmeal
Ingredients:
- 1/2 cup rolled oats
- 1 cup water or milk (almond milk, soy milk, or regular milk)
- 1/4 cup dried cherries
- 2 tablespoons chopped almonds
- Pinch of salt (optional)
- Toppings: Fresh cherries, almond slices, drizzle of honey (optional)

Preparation Method:
1. In a small saucepan, bring the water or milk to a gentle boil over medium heat.
2. Stir in the rolled oats, dried cherries, chopped almonds, and salt (if using).
3. Reduce the heat to low and simmer, stirring occasionally, for about 5-7 minutes or until the oats are tender and the mixture thickens.
4. Once the oats are cooked, remove the saucepan from the heat.
5. Transfer the cherry almond oatmeal to a serving bowl.
6. Top with fresh cherries, almond slices, and a drizzle of honey if desired.
7. Serve warm and enjoy your comforting cherry almond oatmeal.

Tropical Oatmeal
Ingredients:
- 1/2 cup rolled oats
- 1 cup water or milk (almond milk, soy milk, or regular milk)
- 1/4 cup diced pineapple
- 1/4 cup sliced banana
- 2 tablespoons shredded coconut
- Pinch of salt (optional)
- Toppings: Additional diced pineapple, sliced banana, shredded coconut (optional)

Preparation Method:
1. Follow the same preparation method as for basic oatmeal (see previous recipe).
2. When the oatmeal is almost done cooking, stir in the diced pineapple, sliced banana, and shredded coconut.
3. Continue to cook for an additional 1-2 minutes until the mixture is heated through and well combined.
4. Remove from heat and transfer the tropical oatmeal to a serving bowl.
5. Top with additional diced pineapple, sliced banana, and shredded coconut if desired.
6. Serve warm and enjoy your refreshing tropical oatmeal.

Date and Walnut Oatmeal
Ingredients:
- 1/2 cup rolled oats

- 1 cup water or milk (almond milk, soy milk, or regular milk)
- 1/4 cup chopped dates
- 2 tablespoons chopped walnuts
- Pinch of salt (optional)
- Toppings: Sliced dates, chopped walnuts, drizzle of maple syrup (optional)

Preparation Method:
1. Follow the same preparation method as for basic oatmeal (see previous recipe).
2. When the oatmeal is almost done cooking, stir in the chopped dates and chopped walnuts.
3. Continue to cook for an additional 1-2 minutes until the mixture is heated through and well combined.
4. Remove from heat and transfer the date and walnut oatmeal to a serving bowl.
5. Top with sliced dates, chopped walnuts, and a drizzle of maple syrup if desired.
6. Serve warm and enjoy your delicious date and walnut oatmeal.

Maple Pecan Oatmeal
Ingredients:
- 1/2 cup rolled oats
- 1 cup water or milk (almond milk, soy milk, or regular milk)
- 2 tablespoons chopped pecans
- 1-2 tablespoons maple syrup
- Pinch of salt (optional)

- Toppings: Additional chopped pecans, drizzle of maple syrup (optional)

Preparation Method:
1. Follow the same preparation method as for basic oatmeal (see previous recipe).
2. When the oatmeal is almost done cooking, stir in the chopped pecans and maple syrup.
3. Continue to cook for an additional 1-2 minutes until the mixture is heated through and well combined.
4. Remove from heat and transfer the maple pecan oatmeal to a serving bowl.
5. Top with additional chopped pecans and a drizzle of maple syrup if desired.
6. Serve warm and enjoy your delightful maple pecan oatmeal.

Cranberry Orange Oatmeal
Ingredients:
- 1/2 cup rolled oats
- 1 cup water or milk (almond milk, soy milk, or regular milk)
- 2 tablespoons dried cranberries
- Zest of 1 orange
- Pinch of salt (optional)
- Toppings: Fresh orange segments, additional dried cranberries, honey or maple syrup (optional)

Preparation Method:
1. In a small saucepan, bring the water or milk to a gentle boil over medium heat.

2. Stir in the rolled oats, dried cranberries, orange zest, and salt (if using).

3. Reduce the heat to low and simmer, stirring occasionally, for about 5-7 minutes or until the oats are tender and the mixture thickens.

4. Once the oats are cooked, remove the saucepan from the heat.

5. Transfer the cranberry orange oatmeal to a serving bowl.

6. Top with fresh orange segments, additional dried cranberries, and a drizzle of honey or maple syrup if desired.

7. Serve warm and enjoy your delightful cranberry orange oatmeal.

Carrot Cake Oatmeal
Ingredients:
- 1/2 cup rolled oats
- 1 cup water or milk (almond milk, soy milk, or regular milk)
- 1/4 cup grated carrot
- 2 tablespoons chopped walnuts or pecans
- 1/2 teaspoon ground cinnamon
- Pinch of salt (optional)
- Toppings: Shredded coconut, chopped nuts, drizzle of honey or maple syrup (optional)

Preparation Method:
1. Follow the same preparation method as for basic oatmeal (see previous recipe).

2. When the oatmeal is almost done cooking, stir in the grated carrot, chopped nuts, and ground cinnamon.

3. Continue to cook for an additional 1-2 minutes until the carrot is tender.

4. Remove from heat and transfer the carrot cake oatmeal to a serving bowl.

5. Top with shredded coconut, additional chopped nuts, and a drizzle of honey or maple syrup if desired.

6. Serve warm and enjoy your delicious carrot cake oatmeal.

Gingerbread Oatmeal

Ingredients:

- 1/2 cup rolled oats

- 1 cup water or milk (almond milk, soy milk, or regular milk)

- 1 tablespoon molasses

- 1/2 teaspoon ground ginger

- 1/4 teaspoon ground cinnamon

- Pinch of salt (optional)

- Toppings: Chopped nuts, raisins, sprinkle of cinnamon (optional)

Preparation Method:

1. Follow the same preparation method as for basic oatmeal (see previous recipe).

2. When the oatmeal is almost done cooking, stir in the molasses, ground ginger, and ground cinnamon.

3. Continue to cook for an additional 1-2 minutes until the flavors are well combined.

4. Remove from heat and transfer the gingerbread oatmeal to a serving bowl.

5. Top with chopped nuts, raisins, and a sprinkle of cinnamon if desired.

6. Serve warm and enjoy your comforting gingerbread oatmeal.

Espresso Oatmeal

Ingredients:

- 1/2 cup rolled oats
- 1 cup brewed espresso or strong coffee
- 1/4 cup milk (almond milk, soy milk, or regular milk)
- 1 tablespoon cocoa powder
- Pinch of salt (optional)
- Toppings: Chocolate shavings, sliced bananas, chopped nuts (optional)

Preparation Method:

1. In a small saucepan, combine the brewed espresso (or strong coffee), milk, rolled oats, cocoa powder, and salt (if using).

2. Bring to a simmer on medium heat.

3. Reduce the heat to low and simmer, stirring occasionally, for about 5-7 minutes or until the oats are tender and the mixture thickens.

4. Once the oats are cooked, remove the saucepan from the heat.

5. Transfer the espresso oatmeal to a serving bowl.

6. Top with chocolate shavings, sliced bananas, chopped nuts, or any other desired toppings.

7. Serve warm and enjoy your energizing espresso oatmeal.

Savory Oatmeal with Egg

Ingredients:
- 1/2 cup rolled oats
- 1 cup water or vegetable broth
- Pinch of salt (optional)
- Toppings: Fried or poached egg, sautéed vegetables (spinach, mushrooms, cherry tomatoes), shredded cheese, chopped herbs (optional)

Preparation Method:
1. In a small saucepan, bring the water or vegetable broth to a gentle boil over medium heat.
2. Stir in the rolled oats and salt (if using).
3. Reduce the heat to low and simmer, stirring occasionally, for about 5-7 minutes or until the oats are tender and the mixture thickens.
4. While the oats are cooking, prepare your toppings.
5. Once the oats are cooked, remove the saucepan from the heat.
6. Transfer the savory oatmeal to a serving bowl.
7. Top with a fried or poached egg, sautéed vegetables, shredded cheese, chopped herbs, or any other desired toppings.
8. Serve warm and enjoy your satisfying savory oatmeal.

These oatmeal variations offer a range of flavors and textures while being gentle on the digestive system for individuals without a gallbladder. Adjust ingredients and sweetness levels according to personal preferences and dietary restrictions.

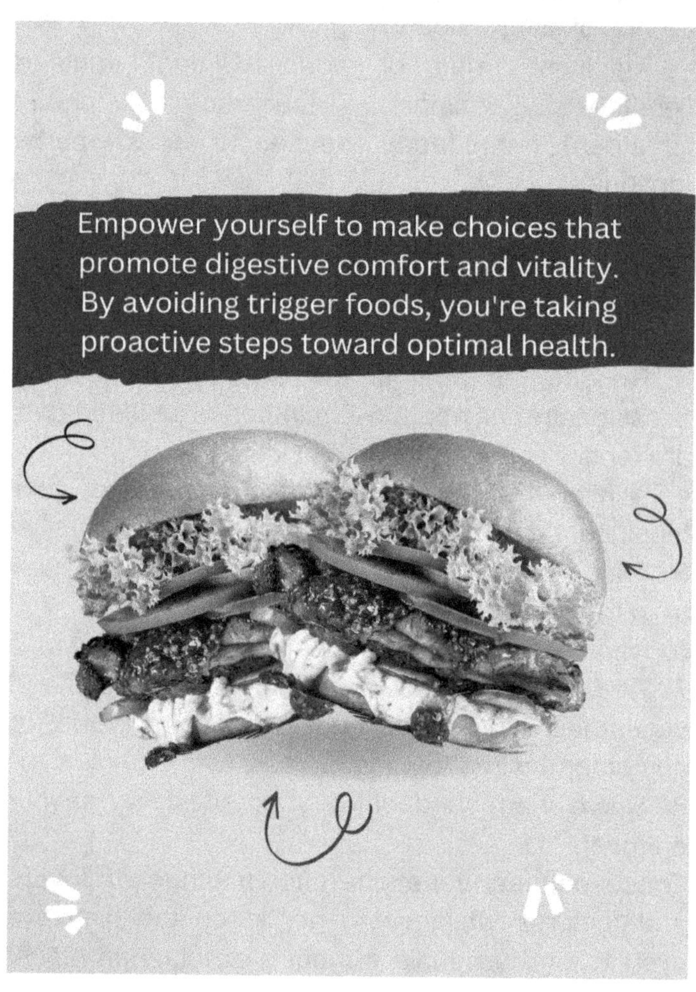

Empower yourself to make choices that promote digestive comfort and vitality. By avoiding trigger foods, you're taking proactive steps toward optimal health.

CHAPTER FIVE

Lunch and Dinner Recipes

When planning lunch and dinner recipes for individuals who have had their gallbladders removed or are following a no-gallbladder diet, it's important to focus on meals that are low in fat, high in fiber, and easily digestible.
Here are some comprehensive lunch and dinner recipes tailored for a no-gallbladder patient:

Flavorful Salad Creations

Certainly! Here are 100 flavorful salad creations suitable for individuals without a gallbladder:

1. Greek Salad
   Ingredients: Cucumber, tomato, red onion, Kalamata olives, feta cheese, oregano, olive oil, lemon juice.

2. Garden Salad
   Ingredients: Mixed greens, cucumber, carrot, tomato, bell pepper, red onion, balsamic vinaigrette.

3. Caesar Salad

Ingredients: Caesar dressing, Parmesan cheese, croutons, and romaine lettuce.

4. Caprese Salad

Ingredients: Tomato, fresh mozzarella, basil leaves, balsamic glaze, olive oil, salt, pepper.

5. Cobb Salad

Ingredients: Mixed greens, grilled chicken, avocado, hard-boiled egg, bacon, blue cheese, ranch dressing.

6. Spinach and Strawberry Salad

Ingredients: Baby spinach, strawberries, goat cheese, almonds, balsamic vinaigrette.

7. Waldorf Salad

Ingredients: Apple, celery, grapes, walnuts, Greek yogurt, honey.

8. Taco Salad

Ingredients: Romaine lettuce, ground turkey or beef, black beans, corn, avocado, salsa, tortilla strips.

9. Mediterranean Quinoa Salad

Ingredients: Quinoa, cucumber, cherry tomatoes, red onion, olives, feta cheese, lemon vinaigrette.

10. Asian Sesame Chicken Salad
Ingredients: Mixed greens, grilled chicken, mandarin oranges, almonds, sesame seeds, sesame ginger dressing.

11. Shrimp and Avocado Salad
Ingredients: Shrimp, avocado, mixed greens, cherry tomatoes, cucumber, lime vinaigrette.

12. Kale Caesar Salad
Ingredients: Kale, croutons, Parmesan cheese, Caesar dressing.

13. Beet and Goat Cheese Salad
Ingredients: Roasted beets, mixed greens, goat cheese, walnuts, balsamic vinaigrette.

14. Apple Pecan Salad
Ingredients: Mixed greens, apple slices, pecans, dried cranberries, blue cheese, apple cider vinaigrette.

15. Tuna Nicoise Salad

Ingredients: Mixed greens, seared tuna, boiled potatoes, green beans, cherry tomatoes, hard-boiled egg, olives, Dijon vinaigrette.

16. Mango Avocado Salad

Ingredients: Mixed greens, mango, avocado, red onion, cilantro, lime vinaigrette.

17. Caesar Pasta Salad

Ingredients: Rotini pasta, Caesar dressing, cherry tomatoes, black olives, Parmesan cheese, croutons.

18. Southwest Chicken Salad

Ingredients: Mixed greens, grilled chicken, black beans, corn, avocado, tomato, cilantro lime dressing.

19. Watermelon Feta Salad

Ingredients: Watermelon cubes, feta cheese, arugula, mint, balsamic glaze.

20. Pear and Walnut Salad

Ingredients: Mixed greens, sliced pear, walnuts, blue cheese, balsamic vinaigrette.

21. Asian Noodle Salad

Ingredients: Rice noodles, mixed vegetables (bell peppers, carrots, cucumber), edamame, sesame ginger dressing.

22. Strawberry Spinach Salad

Ingredients: Baby spinach, sliced strawberries, goat cheese, almonds, balsamic vinaigrette.

23. Chicken Caesar Pasta Salad

Ingredients: Rotini pasta, grilled chicken, Caesar dressing, cherry tomatoes, Parmesan cheese.

24. Quinoa Black Bean Salad

Ingredients: Quinoa, black beans, corn, red bell pepper, cilantro, lime vinaigrette.

25. Mediterranean Chickpea Salad

Ingredients: Chickpeas, cucumber, cherry tomatoes, red onion, feta cheese, Greek dressing.

26. Thai Beef Salad

Ingredients: Thinly sliced beef, mixed greens, cucumber, red onion, cherry tomatoes, cilantro, Thai dressing.

27. Zucchini Ribbon Salad

Ingredients: Zucchini ribbons, cherry tomatoes, basil leaves, mozzarella balls, balsamic vinaigrette.

28. Broccoli Cranberry Salad

Ingredients: Broccoli florets, dried cranberries, sunflower seeds, red onion, Greek yogurt dressing.

29. Mediterranean Orzo Salad

Ingredients: Orzo pasta, cucumber, cherry tomatoes, olives, feta cheese, lemon vinaigrette.

30. Caesar Wedge Salad

Ingredients: Iceberg lettuce wedge, bacon bits, cherry tomatoes, blue cheese dressing.

31. Kale Apple Salad

Ingredients: Kale, apple slices, pecans, goat cheese, apple cider vinaigrette.

32. Mango Black Bean Salad

Ingredients: Mango, black beans, red bell pepper, red onion, cilantro, lime vinaigrette.

33. Italian Pasta Salad

Ingredients: Rotini pasta, cherry tomatoes, black olives, mozzarella balls, Italian dressing.

34. Grilled Vegetable Salad

Ingredients: Grilled zucchini, bell peppers, eggplant, red onion, mixed greens, balsamic vinaigrette.

35. Asian Cucumber Salad

Ingredients: Thinly sliced cucumber, sesame seeds, green onions, rice vinegar dressing.

36. Antipasto Salad

Ingredients: Salami, pepperoni, mozzarella cheese, olives, roasted red peppers, Italian dressing.

37. Potato Salad

Ingredients: Boiled potatoes, celery, red onion, pickles, Greek yogurt dressing.

38. Arugula Strawberry Salad

Ingredients: Arugula, sliced strawberries, goat cheese, almonds, balsamic vinaigrette.

39. Greek Couscous Salad

Ingredients: Couscous, cucumber, cherry tomatoes, feta cheese, olives, Greek dressing.

40. Southwest Quinoa Salad

Ingredients: Quinoa, black beans, corn, bell peppers, avocado, lime vinaigrette.

41. Spinach Walnut Salad

Ingredients: Baby spinach, chopped walnuts, dried cranberries, feta cheese, balsamic vinaigrette.

42. Tabbouleh Salad

Ingredients: Bulgur wheat, parsley, tomatoes, cucumber, red onion, lemon dressing.

43. Asian Slaw Salad

Ingredients: Shredded cabbage, carrots, bell peppers, green onions, sesame ginger dressing.

44. Pear Gorgonzola Salad

Ingredients: Mixed greens, sliced pears, gorgonzola cheese, candied pecans, balsamic vinaigrette.

45. Orzo Pesto Salad

Ingredients: Orzo pasta, cherry tomatoes, mozzarella balls, pesto dressing.

46. Broccoli Bacon Salad

Ingredients: Broccoli florets, bacon bits, sunflower seeds, red onion, Greek yogurt dressing.

47. Spring Mix Salad
Ingredients: Spring mix greens, avocado, cherry tomatoes, cucumber, lemon vinaigrette.

48. Shrimp Mango Salad
Ingredients: Grilled shrimp, mango chunks, mixed greens, avocado, lime vinaigrette.

49. Radicchio Orange Salad
Ingredients: Radicchio leaves, orange segments, fennel, almonds, citrus dressing.

50. Asian Cabbage Salad
Ingredients: Shredded cabbage, mandarin oranges, sliced almonds, sesame seeds, soy ginger dressing.

51. Egg Salad
Ingredients: Hard-boiled eggs, mixed greens, cherry tomatoes, cucumber, honey mustard dressing.

52. Avocado Corn Salad
Ingredients: Corn kernels, avocado chunks, cherry tomatoes, cilantro, lime vinaigrette.

53. Chickpea Avocado Salad

Ingredients: Chickpeas, avocado, cherry tomatoes, red onion, cilantro, lime vinaigrette.

54. Summer Berry Salad

Ingredients: Mixed greens, raspberries, blueberries, blackberries, goat cheese, raspberry vinaigrette.

55. Artichoke Heart Salad

Ingredients: Artichoke hearts, roasted red peppers, cherry tomatoes, Kalamata olives, Italian dressing.

56. Quinoa Arugula Salad

Ingredients: Quinoa, arugula, cherry tomatoes, cucumber, feta cheese, lemon vinaigrette.

57. Cranberry Walnut Spinach Salad

Ingredients: Baby spinach, dried cranberries, chopped walnuts, red onion, raspberry vinaigrette.

58. Edamame Salad

Ingredients: Edamame beans, red bell pepper, carrot, green onions, sesame ginger dressing.

59. Three Bean Salad
Ingredients: Kidney beans, black beans, green beans, red onion, Italian dressing.

60. Avocado Tomato Salad
Ingredients: Avocado, cherry tomatoes, red onion, cilantro, lime vinaigrette.

61. Roasted Beet Salad
Ingredients: Roasted beets, mixed greens, goat cheese, candied walnuts, balsamic vinaigrette.

62. Lemon Herb Quinoa Salad
Ingredients: Quinoa, cucumber, cherry tomatoes, fresh herbs (parsley, mint, dill), lemon dressing.

63. Fennel Orange Salad
Ingredients: Fennel bulb, orange segments, arugula, almonds, citrus dressing.

64. Spicy Mango Cucumber Salad
Ingredients: Mango, cucumber, red chili flakes, lime juice, cilantro.

65. Corn Tomato Avocado Salad

Ingredients: Corn kernels, cherry tomatoes, avocado, red onion, lime vinaigrette.

66. Italian Chopped Salad

Ingredients: Romaine lettuce, salami, provolone cheese, cherry tomatoes, red onion, Italian dressing.

67. Apple Walnut Salad

Ingredients: Mixed greens, apple slices, chopped walnuts, blue cheese, apple cider vinaigrette.

68. Mexican Street Corn Salad

Ingredients: Grilled corn, cotija cheese, chili powder, lime juice, cilantro.

69. Lemon Kale Salad

Ingredients: Kale, lemon zest, parmesan cheese, toasted breadcrumbs, lemon vinaigrette.

70. Grilled Chicken Mango Salad

Ingredients: Grilled chicken, mango slices, mixed greens, avocado, lime vinaigrette.

71. Broccoli Quinoa Salad

Ingredients: Quinoa, broccoli florets, cherry tomatoes, red onion, lemon vinaigrette.

72. Asian Pear Salad

Ingredients: Mixed greens, Asian pear slices, candied pecans, blue cheese, ginger dressing.

73. Lentil Cucumber Salad

Ingredients: Cooked lentils, cucumber, cherry tomatoes, red onion, parsley, lemon dressing.

74. Radish Cucumber Salad

Ingredients: Radishes, cucumber, red onion, dill, Greek yogurt dressing.

75. Blue Cheese Pear Salad

Ingredients: Mixed greens, sliced pears, blue cheese crumbles, pecans, balsamic vinaigrette.

76. Melon Prosciutto Salad

Ingredients: Melon balls, prosciutto slices, arugula, balsamic glaze.

77. Thai Papaya Salad

Ingredients: Shredded green papaya, cherry tomatoes, peanuts, Thai dressing.

78. Broccoli Apple Salad

Ingredients: Broccoli florets, apple chunks, raisins, sunflower seeds, Greek yogurt dressing.

79. Avocado Egg Salad

Ingredients: Hard-boiled eggs, avocado, mixed greens, cherry tomatoes, balsamic vinaigrette.

80. Spicy Peanut Noodle Salad

Ingredients: Rice noodles, bell peppers, carrots, cilantro, peanut dressing.

81. Cauliflower Tabouli Salad

Ingredients: Cauliflower rice, parsley, cherry tomatoes, cucumber, lemon dressing.

82. Orange Almond Salad

Ingredients: Mixed greens, orange segments, sliced almonds, feta cheese, citrus dressing.

83. Tomato Basil Mozzarella Salad

Ingredients: Cherry tomatoes, fresh mozzarella balls, basil leaves, balsamic glaze.

84. Cranberry Spinach Salad

Ingredients: Baby spinach, dried cranberries, goat cheese, pecans, balsamic vinaigrette.

85. Pomegranate Walnut

86. Pomegranate Walnut Salad
Ingredients: Mixed greens, pomegranate seeds, walnuts, feta cheese, balsamic vinaigrette.

87. Citrus Avocado Salad
Ingredients: Mixed greens, orange segments, avocado slices, red onion, citrus vinaigrette.

88. Cranberry Kale Salad
Ingredients: Kale, dried cranberries, pumpkin seeds, feta cheese, apple cider vinaigrette.

89. Radish Apple Salad
Ingredients: Radishes, apple slices, arugula, almonds, lemon vinaigrette.

90. Pear Walnut Gorgonzola Salad
Ingredients: Mixed greens, sliced pears, walnuts, gorgonzola cheese, balsamic vinaigrette.

91. Grilled Peach Salad

Ingredients: Grilled peaches, mixed greens, goat cheese, almonds, honey balsamic dressing.

92. Quinoa Spinach Salad

Ingredients: Quinoa, baby spinach, cherry tomatoes, cucumber, feta cheese, lemon vinaigrette.

93. Mango Jalapeno Salad

Ingredients: Mixed greens, mango chunks, jalapeno slices, red onion, lime vinaigrette.

94. Cucumber Tomato Salad

Ingredients: Sliced cucumbers, cherry tomatoes, red onion, dill, red wine vinaigrette.

95. Tzatziki Cucumber Salad

Ingredients: Sliced cucumbers, cherry tomatoes, red onion, tzatziki sauce.

96. Beet Goat Cheese Salad

Ingredients: Roasted beets, mixed greens, goat cheese, walnuts, balsamic vinaigrette.

97. Strawberry Poppy Seed Salad

Ingredients: Mixed greens, sliced strawberries, goat cheese, almonds, poppy seed dressing.

98. Pineapple Cucumber Salad

Ingredients: Diced pineapple, sliced cucumbers, red bell pepper, cilantro, lime dressing.

99. Mango Black Bean Quinoa Salad

Ingredients: Quinoa, black beans, mango chunks, red bell pepper, cilantro lime dressing.

100. Mixed Berry Spinach Salad

Ingredients: Baby spinach, mixed berries (strawberries, blueberries, raspberries), pecans, raspberry vinaigrette.

These salads offer a variety of flavors, textures, and nutrients, making them delicious and satisfying options for individuals without a gallbladder. Adjust the ingredients and dressings according to personal preferences and dietary needs.

Light Soups

Here's a list of 100 light soup ideas suitable for individuals without a gallbladder:

1. Vegetable Broth Soup
2. Chicken and Rice Soup
3. Lentil Soup

4. Tomato Basil Soup
5. Miso Soup
6. Spinach and White Bean Soup
7. Butternut Squash Soup
8. Carrot Ginger Soup
9. Chicken Noodle Soup
10. Minestrone Soup
11. Cauliflower Soup
12. Potato Leek Soup
13. Broccoli Cheddar Soup (with low-fat cheese)
14. Turkey Meatball Soup
15. Mushroom Barley Soup
16. Zucchini Soup
17. Sweet Potato Soup
18. Quinoa Vegetable Soup
19. Cabbage Soup
20. Navy Bean Soup
21. Thai Coconut Soup (with light coconut milk)
22. Lemon Chicken Orzo Soup
23. Egg Drop Soup
24. Gazpacho
25. Green Pea Soup
26. Asparagus Soup
27. Beet Soup
28. Corn Chowder (with skim milk)
29. Chicken Tortilla Soup
30. Pasta Fagioli Soup
31. Artichoke Soup
32. Black Bean Soup
33. Turkey Vegetable Soup
34. Split Pea Soup
35. Roasted Red Pepper Soup

36. Chicken and Wild Rice Soup
37. Escarole Soup
38. Barley Vegetable Soup
39. Spicy Pumpkin Soup
40. Cauliflower and Cheese Soup (with low-fat cheese)
41. Italian Wedding Soup
42. Broccoli Soup
43. Lentil and Kale Soup
44. Green Bean Soup
45. Chickpea Soup
46. Moroccan Lentil Soup
47. Creamy Mushroom Soup (with low-fat milk)
48. Rice and Vegetable Soup
49. Brussels Sprouts Soup
50. Chicken and Vegetable Soup
51. Spinach Egg Drop Soup
52. Leek and Potato Soup
53. Pea and Mint Soup
54. Tomato Egg Drop Soup
55. Tomato Orzo Soup
56. Cucumber Soup
57. Carrot Soup
58. Chicken and Barley Soup
59. Tomato Spinach Soup
60. Swiss Chard Soup
61. White Bean and Kale Soup
62. Spinach and Lentil Soup
63. Chicken and Corn Soup
64. Chickpea and Spinach Soup
65. Artichoke and Spinach Soup
66. Quinoa and Vegetable Soup

67. Green Lentil Soup
68. Creamy Asparagus Soup
69. Mushroom Soup
70. White Bean and Escarole Soup
71. Turkey and Vegetable Soup
72. Lemon Rice Soup
73. Beef and Vegetable Soup (with lean beef)
74. Lima Bean Soup
75. Eggplant Soup
76. Cabbage and Potato Soup
77. Celery Soup
78. Fennel Soup
79. Swiss Chard and White Bean Soup
80. Chicken and Cabbage Soup
81. Cucumber Avocado Soup
82. Lemon Chickpea Soup
83. Turkey Chili
84. White Bean and Tomato Soup
85. Kale and Quinoa Soup
86. Chicken and Mushroom Soup
87. Farro and Vegetable Soup
88. Rice and Lentil Soup
89. Turkey and Black Bean Soup
90. Lemon Lentil Soup
91. Parsnip Soup
92. Turnip Soup
93. Chicken and Farro Soup
94. Spring Vegetable Soup
95. Cauliflower and Chickpea Soup
96. Spaghetti Squash Soup
97. Chicken and Edamame Soup
98. Navy Bean and Spinach Soup

99. Chicken and Cabbage Soup
100. Quinoa and Black Bean Soup

These soup options are light, nutritious, and suitable for individuals without a gallbladder. Adjust ingredients and seasonings according to personal preferences and dietary needs.

Delicious Stews

Variety of stew ideas that you can adapt to suit the preferences and dietary needs of individuals without a gallbladder.
Here are some stew ideas:

1. Chicken and Vegetable Stew
2. Beef and Barley Stew
3. Lentil and Potato Stew
4. Turkey and Quinoa Stew
5. Vegetable Bean Stew
6. Fish Stew with Tomatoes and Olives
7. Moroccan Chickpea Stew
8. Italian Sausage and White Bean Stew
9. Mushroom and Wild Rice Stew
10. Butternut Squash and Lentil Stew
11. Chicken and Sweet Potato Stew
12. Beef and Vegetable Stew
13. Spicy Black Bean Stew
14. Thai Coconut Vegetable Stew
15. Lamb and Chickpea Stew
16. Ratatouille Stew
17. Turkey and Mushroom Stew

18. Root Vegetable Stew
19. Mediterranean Fish Stew
20. Curried Lentil Stew
21. Chicken and White Bean Stew
22. Beef and Mushroom Stew
23. Potato and Leek Stew
24. Vegetable Quinoa Stew
25. Mexican Chicken Stew
26. Seafood Stew with Fennel and Tomatoes
27. Irish Beef and Guinness Stew
28. Moroccan Lamb Stew with Apricots
29. Tuscan White Bean and Kale Stew
30. Cajun Shrimp and Sausage Stew
31. Chicken and Wild Rice Stew
32. Vegetarian Chili Stew
33. Hungarian Goulash Stew
34. Beef and Cabbage Stew
35. Portuguese Fish Stew
36. Chicken and Corn Stew
37. Moroccan Vegetable Stew
38. Italian Wedding Soup Stew
39. Turkey and Black Bean Stew
40. Sweet Potato and Black Bean Stew
41. Beef and Lentil Stew
42. Vegetable and Chickpea Stew
43. French Onion Soup Stew
44. Chicken and Chickpea Stew
45. Caribbean Fish Stew
46. Italian Tomato and Vegetable Stew
47. Beef and Potato Stew
48. Chicken and Rice Stew
49. Lentil and Kale Stew

50. Thai Peanut Chicken Stew

These stew ideas provide a starting point, and you can experiment with different combinations of meats, vegetables, legumes, and seasonings to create flavorful and nutritious dishes for individuals without a gallbladder. Adjust ingredients and seasonings according to personal preferences and dietary restrictions.

Grilled and Baked Entrées

Certainly! Here's a list of 100 grilled and baked entrées suitable for individuals without a gallbladder:

Grilled Entrées

1. Grilled Chicken Breast
2. Grilled Salmon Fillet
3. Grilled Turkey Burger
4. Grilled Shrimp Skewers
5. Grilled Vegetable Platter
6. Grilled Pork Chops
7. Grilled Tofu Steaks
8. Grilled Swordfish Steak
9. Grilled Portobello Mushrooms
10. Grilled Lamb Chops
11. Grilled Veggie Kebabs
12. Grilled Mahi Mahi Fillet
13. Grilled Turkey Breast
14. Grilled Halibut Steak

15. Grilled Veggie Burgers
16. Grilled Ribeye Steak
17. Grilled Chicken Skewers
18. Grilled Tilapia Fillet
19. Grilled Eggplant Slices
20. Grilled Flank Steak
21. Grilled Sea Bass Fillet
22. Grilled Veggie Quesadillas
23. Grilled Tuna Steak
24. Grilled Asparagus Spears
25. Grilled Bison Burger
26. Grilled Cod Fillet
27. Grilled Halloumi Cheese
28. Grilled Zucchini Slices
29. Grilled Turkey Sausages
30. Grilled Octopus Tentacles
31. Grilled Corn on the Cob
32. Grilled Chicken Thighs
33. Grilled Trout Fillet
34. Grilled Stuffed Bell Peppers
35. Grilled Sirloin Steak
36. Grilled Scallops
37. Grilled Pineapple Rings
38. Grilled Chicken Wings
39. Grilled Catfish Fillet
40. Grilled Sweet Potato Wedges
41. Grilled Lamb Burgers
42. Grilled Haloumi Skewers
43. Grilled Cherry Tomatoes
44. Grilled Quail
45. Grilled Fennel Slices
46. Grilled Bison Ribeye

47. Grilled Crab Legs
48. Grilled Bratwurst Sausages
49. Grilled Polenta Slices
50. Grilled Swordfish Skewers

Baked Entrées

51. Baked Chicken Parmesan
52. Baked Salmon with Dill Sauce
53. Baked Turkey Meatballs
54. Baked Cod with Lemon Herb Crust
55. Baked Eggplant Parmesan
56. Baked Pork Tenderloin
57. Baked Tofu Nuggets
58. Baked Halibut with Garlic Butter
59. Baked Vegetable Lasagna
60. Baked Lamb Meatballs
61. Baked Stuffed Peppers
62. Baked Lemon Herb Chicken
63. Baked Tilapia with Mango Salsa
64. Baked Portobello Mushrooms with Goat Cheese
65. Baked Turkey Meatloaf
66. Baked Mahi Mahi with Pesto Crust
67. Baked Veggie Casserole
68. Baked Ribeye Steak with Mushrooms
69. Baked Chicken Drumsticks
70. Baked Cod with Mediterranean Vegetables
71. Baked Turkey Breast with Cranberry Glaze
72. Baked Flounder with Tomato Basil Sauce
73. Baked Stuffed Zucchini Boats

74. Baked Bison Meatballs
75. Baked Crab Cakes with Remoulade Sauce
76. Baked Chicken Fajitas
77. Baked Trout with Almond Crust
78. Baked Spinach and Feta Stuffed Chicken
79. Baked Swordfish with Tomato Relish
80. Baked Stuffed Mushrooms
81. Baked Turkey Burgers with Avocado
82. Baked Lemon Garlic Shrimp
83. Baked Halibut with Mango Salsa
84. Baked Veggie Stuffed Bell Peppers
85. Baked Lamb Chops with Rosemary
86. Baked Salmon with Honey Mustard Glaze
87. Baked Turkey Chili
88. Baked Cod with Herbed Breadcrumbs
89. Baked Eggplant Rollatini
90. Baked Bison Burgers with Caramelized Onions
91. Baked Tilapia with Parmesan Crust
92. Baked Stuffed Cabbage Rolls
93. Baked Lemon Herb Halibut
94. Baked Chicken Alfredo Pasta
95. Baked Stuffed Artichokes
96. Baked Turkey and Vegetable Casserole
97. Baked Salmon with Garlic Butter
98. Baked Portobello Mushroom Caps with Brie
99. Baked Lamb Shanks
100. Baked Stuffed Squash

These grilled and baked entrées offer a variety of protein options and flavors for individuals without a gallbladder. Adjust seasonings and accompaniments according to personal preferences and dietary restrictions.

CHAPTER FIVE

Snacks and Appetizers

Snacks and appetizers play a significant role in maintaining energy levels and satisfying hunger between meals for individuals without a gallbladder. These options should be low in fat, easily digestible, and ideally rich in nutrients.

Healthy Snacks

Here's a list of healthy snacks suitable for individuals without a gallbladder:

1. Apple slices with almond butter
2. Carrot sticks with hummus
3. Greek yogurt with berries
4. Celery sticks with peanut butter
5. Cottage cheese with pineapple chunks
6. Whole grain crackers with cheese slices
7. Trail mix with nuts and dried fruits
8. Rice cakes with avocado slices
9. Edamame beans
10. Hard-boiled eggs
11. Cherry tomatoes with mozzarella balls
12. Almonds
13. Banana slices with peanut butter
14. Popcorn (air-popped)
15. Cucumber slices with tzatziki
16. Bell pepper strips with guacamole

17. Kale chips
18. Roasted chickpeas
19. Sliced turkey breast roll-ups with lettuce and mustard
20. Mixed nuts (unsalted)
21. Apple slices with cinnamon
22. Cottage cheese with sliced strawberries
23. Veggie sticks with yogurt dip
24. Rice cakes with cottage cheese and tomato slices
25. Greek yogurt with honey and granola
26. Seaweed snacks
27. Frozen grapes
28. Almond and date energy balls
29. Pumpkin seeds
30. Sliced pear with ricotta cheese
31. Whole grain toast with mashed avocado
32. Baby carrots with tahini
33. Turkey jerky
34. Berries with cottage cheese
35. Sunflower seeds
36. Dried apricots
37. Whole grain crackers with tuna salad
38. Rice cakes with almond butter and banana slices
39. Cottage cheese with diced peaches
40. Snap peas
41. Cherry tomatoes with cottage cheese
42. Apple slices with cottage cheese
43. Greek yogurt with sliced almonds
44. Celery sticks with cream cheese
45. Hard-boiled eggs with mustard

46. Seaweed salad
47. Popcorn with nutritional yeast
48. Cucumber slices with cream cheese and smoked salmon
49. Rice cakes with sliced turkey breast
50. Mixed berries with Greek yogurt
51. Trail mix with dark chocolate chips
52. Greek yogurt with sliced kiwi
53. Almond butter on rice cakes
54. Cottage cheese with pineapple and walnuts
55. Carrot sticks with yogurt dip
56. Cherry tomatoes with balsamic glaze
57. Sliced turkey breast with cucumber slices
58. Greek yogurt with chia seeds and honey
59. Rice cakes with mashed avocado and tomato slices
60. Popcorn with cinnamon
61. Almonds with dried cranberries
62. Sliced apple with cottage cheese and cinnamon
63. Celery sticks with almond butter and raisins
64. Greek yogurt with sliced strawberries
65. Whole grain crackers with tuna and avocado
66. Turkey roll-ups with cream cheese and cucumber
67. Bell pepper strips with salsa
68. Cottage cheese with sliced grapes
69. Edamame hummus with veggie sticks
70. Rice cakes with sliced cucumber and hummus
71. Greek yogurt with sliced peaches
72. Almond butter on apple slices
73. Hard-boiled eggs with avocado
74. Trail mix with pumpkin seeds

75. Cottage cheese with mandarin orange segments
76. Carrot sticks with tzatziki
77. Sliced turkey breast with mustard
78. Greek yogurt with blueberries
79. Rice cakes with cottage cheese and pineapple chunks
80. Popcorn with Parmesan cheese
81. Mixed nuts with dried cherries
82. Sliced apple with almond butter
83. Celery sticks with tuna salad
84. Greek yogurt with mango slices
85. Rice cakes with almond butter and honey
86. Cottage cheese with diced pear
87. Bell pepper strips with hummus
88. Turkey roll-ups with cream cheese and olives
89. Edamame with sea salt
90. Popcorn with chili powder
91. Sliced cucumber with cottage cheese and pepper
92. Greek yogurt with raspberries
93. Almond butter on banana slices
94. Hard-boiled eggs with hot sauce
95. Trail mix with cashews
96. Cottage cheese with kiwi slices
97. Carrot sticks with guacamole
98. Sliced turkey breast with cream cheese
99. Greek yogurt with sliced banana
100. Rice cakes with tuna salad
101. Popcorn with garlic powder
102. Mixed nuts with dried apricots
103. Sliced apple with peanut butter

104. Celery sticks with almond butter and dried cranberries
105. Greek yogurt with pineapple chunks
106. Rice cakes with cottage cheese and sliced strawberries
107. Cottage cheese with mango chunks
108. Bell pepper strips with Greek yogurt dip
109. Turkey roll-ups with cream cheese and bell pepper slices
110. Edamame with soy sauce
111. Popcorn with rosemary
112. Sliced cucumber with hummus
113. Greek yogurt with blackberries
114. Almond butter on celery sticks
115. Hard-boiled eggs with salsa
116. Trail mix with almonds
117. Cottage cheese with banana slices
118. Carrot sticks with beet hummus
119. Sliced turkey breast with avocado
120. Greek yogurt with orange segments
121. Rice cakes with almond butter and sliced strawberries
122. Popcorn with cayenne pepper
123. Mixed nuts with dried mango
124. Sliced apple with cottage cheese and honey
125. Celery sticks with peanut butter and raisins
126. Greek yogurt with mixed berries
127. Almond butter on rice cakes with banana slices
128. Cottage cheese with melon chunks
129. Bell pepper strips with avocado dip

130. Turkey roll-ups with cream cheese and cucumber slices
131. Edamame with chili flakes
132. Popcorn with nutritional yeast and garlic powder
133. Sliced cucumber with cream cheese and smoked salmon
134. Greek yogurt with sliced kiwi and granola
135. Rice cakes with hummus and cucumber slices
136. Cottage cheese with peach slices
137. Carrot sticks with Greek yogurt dip
138. Sliced turkey breast with cream cheese and cucumber slices
139. Greek yogurt with sliced strawberries and granola
140. Almond butter on apple slices with cinnamon
141. Hard-boiled eggs with guacamole
142. Trail mix with walnuts
143. Cottage cheese with raspberry compote
144. Popcorn with turmeric
145. Mixed nuts with dried blueberries
146. Sliced apple with almond butter and raisins
147. Celery sticks with hummus and sunflower seeds
148. Greek yogurt with mango chunks and shredded coconut
149. Rice cakes with avocado and tomato slices
150. Cottage cheese with pear slices and cinnamon
151. Carrot sticks with tzatziki and olives
152. Sliced turkey breast with cream cheese and bell pepper strips
153. Greek yogurt with sliced peach and almonds

154. Rice cakes with cottage cheese and mango chunks
155. Popcorn with paprika
156. Mixed nuts with dried pineapple
157. Sliced cucumber with hummus and cherry tomatoes
158. Greek yogurt with sliced apple and cinnamon
159. Almond butter on banana slices with chia seeds
160. Hard-boiled eggs with pesto
161. Carrot sticks with cilantro yogurt dip
162. Sliced turkey breast with cucumber slices and mustard
163. Greek yogurt with sliced mango and pistachios
164. Rice cakes with hummus and sliced radishes
165. Cottage cheese with mixed berries and honey
166. Bell pepper strips with Greek yogurt ranch dip
167. Turkey roll-ups with cream cheese and spinach leaves
168. Edamame with sesame seeds
169. Popcorn with lemon pepper seasoning
170. Mixed nuts with dried figs
171. Sliced apple with cottage cheese and almonds
172. Celery sticks with peanut butter and dark chocolate chips
173. Greek yogurt with sliced pear and walnuts
174. Rice cakes with almond butter and sliced grapes
175. Cottage cheese with cherry tomatoes and basil
176. Carrot sticks with tzatziki and cucumber slices

177. Sliced turkey breast with cream cheese and avocado slices
178. Greek yogurt with pineapple chunks and macadamia nuts
179. Rice cakes with hummus and roasted red pepper slices
180. Popcorn with Italian seasoning
181. Mixed nuts with dried cranberries and pumpkin seeds
182. Sliced cucumber with hummus and olives
183. Greek yogurt with sliced banana and hemp seeds
184. Almond butter on apple slices with shredded coconut
185. Hard-boiled eggs with sriracha
186. Cottage cheese with grapefruit segments
187. Carrot sticks with avocado hummus
188. Sliced turkey breast with cream cheese and tomato slices
189. Greek yogurt with sliced kiwi and flaxseeds
190. Rice cakes with almond butter and sliced kiwi
191. Popcorn with garlic and herb seasoning
192. Mixed nuts with goji berries
193. Sliced apple with almond butter and sunflower seeds
194. Celery sticks with hummus and cherry tomatoes
195. Greek yogurt with diced mango and pumpkin seeds
196. Rice cakes with cottage cheese and sliced peaches

197. Cottage cheese with blackberries and sliced almonds
198. Carrot sticks with spicy avocado dip
199. Sliced turkey breast with cream cheese and cucumber sticks

These snacks offer a combination of protein, healthy fats, and fiber, making them nutritious options for individuals without a gallbladder. Adjust portion sizes according to personal preferences and dietary needs.

Appetizers

1. Vegetable crudité with hummus
2. Stuffed grape leaves (dolmas)
3. Greek salad skewers
4. Caprese salad bites with cherry tomatoes, mozzarella, and basil
5. Shrimp cocktail with cocktail sauce
6. Deviled eggs with avocado instead of mayo
7. Cucumber slices topped with smoked salmon and cream cheese
8. Spinach and feta phyllo triangles
9. Edamame with sea salt
10. Guacamole with cucumber slices
11. Grilled shrimp skewers
12. Bruschetta with tomato, basil, and balsamic glaze
13. Stuffed mushrooms with spinach and cheese
14. Antipasto platter with olives, cheese, and cured meats

15. Smoked salmon pinwheels with cream cheese
16. Grilled vegetable platter with balsamic glaze
17. Roasted red pepper hummus with pita triangles
18. Cucumber and tomato gazpacho shots
19. Mini turkey meatballs with marinara sauce
20. Crab cakes with lemon aioli
21. Sliced turkey breast wraps with lettuce and mustard
22. Roasted garlic and white bean dip with carrot sticks
23. Chicken skewers with peanut dipping sauce
24. Mini quiches with spinach and feta
25. Sushi rolls with avocado and cucumber
26. Stuffed bell peppers with quinoa and black beans
27. Tuna salad on cucumber rounds
28. Artichoke hearts with lemon aioli
29. Zucchini fritters with yogurt sauce
30. Stuffed cherry tomatoes with herbed goat cheese
31. Caprese skewers with balsamic glaze
32. Roasted chickpeas with spices
33. Beet and goat cheese crostini
34. Smoked salmon on endive leaves with dill cream cheese
35. Grilled asparagus wrapped in prosciutto
36. Mini chicken lettuce wraps
37. Roasted eggplant dip with whole grain crackers
38. Greek yogurt tzatziki with sliced cucumbers
39. Stuffed jalapeno poppers with cream cheese
40. Watermelon and feta skewers with mint
41. Mini crab-stuffed bell peppers

42. Tomato bruschetta with basil and garlic

43. Cucumber cups filled with tuna salad

44. Marinated olives with herbs and citrus zest

45. Spinach and artichoke dip with carrot sticks

46. Smoked trout pate on cucumber slices

47. Chicken satay skewers with peanut sauce

48. Goat cheese and fig crostini

49. Prosciutto-wrapped melon slices

50. Roasted vegetable platter with tahini dip

51. Bacon-wrapped dates stuffed with almonds

52. Smoked salmon and cucumber roll-ups with cream cheese

53. Stuffed avocado halves with shrimp salad

54. Tomato and mozzarella skewers with pesto drizzle

55. Buffalo cauliflower bites with yogurt dipping sauce

56. Shrimp ceviche with avocado

57. Cucumber boats filled with crab salad

58. Stuffed artichoke hearts with breadcrumbs and Parmesan

59. Roasted red pepper and feta dip with pita chips

60. Mini vegetable spring rolls with dipping sauce

61. Endive leaves filled with herbed goat cheese

62. Mini turkey sliders on lettuce wraps

63. Roasted vegetable bruschetta with goat cheese

64. Mediterranean-style stuffed grape leaves

65. Crab and avocado stacks with lime dressing

66. Chicken and vegetable skewers with teriyaki glaze

67. Spinach and cheese stuffed cherry tomatoes

68. Smoked salmon and avocado salad in cucumber cups

69. Beet hummus with carrot sticks

70. Caprese-stuffed portobello mushrooms

71. Grilled shrimp with mango salsa

72. Tomato and basil skewers with balsamic reduction

73. Spicy tuna tartare on crispy wonton chips

74. Greek-style stuffed mushrooms with spinach and feta

75. Cucumber cups filled with Greek yogurt and dill

76. Baked sweet potato fries with yogurt dipping sauce

77. Mini turkey lettuce wraps with hoisin sauce

78. Asparagus wrapped in prosciutto with lemon zest

79. Quinoa-stuffed bell peppers with black beans and corn

80. Smoked salmon and avocado rolls with cream cheese

81. Mediterranean antipasto skewers with olives, cheese, and peppers

82. Chicken avocado roll-ups with salsa

83. Zucchini roll-ups with herbed cream cheese

84. Roasted cauliflower bites with tahini dipping sauce

85. Stuffed cherry peppers with herbed ricotta

86. Bacon-wrapped shrimp with BBQ sauce

87. Cucumber cups filled with smoked salmon mousse

88. Spinach and cheese stuffed mushrooms

89. Greek yogurt dip with assorted vegetable sticks

90. Mini turkey meatballs with marinara dipping sauce
91. Tomato and mozzarella bruschetta with balsamic glaze
92. Shrimp and avocado salad in cucumber boats
93. Caprese skewers with cherry tomatoes, mozzarella, and basil
94. Grilled vegetable platter with hummus
95. Stuffed bell peppers with quinoa and black beans
96. Chicken satay skewers with peanut sauce
97. Smoked salmon pinwheels with herbed cream cheese
98. Greek salad skewers with feta cheese
99. Cucumber slices topped with crab salad
100. Prosciutto-wrapped asparagus spears
101. Roasted red pepper hummus with pita chips
102. Mini turkey sliders on lettuce wraps
103. Grilled shrimp skewers with mango salsa
104. Tomato bruschetta with basil and garlic
105. Stuffed mushrooms with spinach and cheese
106. Deviled eggs with avocado instead of mayo
107. Watermelon and feta skewers with mint
108. Beet hummus with carrot sticks
109. Stuffed cherry tomatoes with herbed goat cheese
110. Bacon-wrapped dates stuffed with almonds
111. Artichoke hearts with lemon aioli
112. Zucchini fritters with yogurt sauce
113. Stuffed jalapeno poppers with cream cheese
114. Smoked salmon on cucumber rounds with dill cream cheese

115. Mini crab-stuffed bell peppers
116. Greek yogurt tzatziki with sliced cucumbers
117. Stuffed avocado halves with shrimp salad
118. Marinated olives with herbs and citrus zest
119. Spinach and artichoke dip with carrot sticks
120. Smoked trout pate on cucumber slices
121. Chicken satay skewers with peanut sauce
122. Goat cheese and fig crostini
123. Prosciutto-wrapped melon slices
124. Roasted vegetable platter with tahini dip
125. Bacon-wrapped dates stuffed with goat cheese
126. Mediterranean-style stuffed grape leaves
127. Crab and avocado stacks with lime dressing
128. Tomato and mozzarella skewers with pesto drizzle
129. Buffalo cauliflower bites with yogurt dipping sauce
130. Shrimp ceviche with avocado
131. Cucumber boats filled with crab salad
132. Stuffed artichoke hearts with breadcrumbs and Parmesan
133. Roasted red pepper
134. Roasted chickpeas with spices
135. Grilled vegetable platter with balsamic glaze
136. Greek yogurt with sliced cucumber and dill
137. Cucumber slices topped with smoked salmon and avocado
138. Caprese salad bites with cherry tomatoes, mozzarella, and basil
139. Stuffed grape leaves (dolmas) with rice and herbs

140. Hummus with carrot and celery sticks
141. Avocado salsa with whole grain tortilla chips
142. Shrimp cocktail with lemon wedges and cocktail sauce
143. Greek yogurt dip with assorted vegetable sticks
144. Edamame beans with sea salt
145. Roasted vegetable bruschetta on whole grain baguette slices
146. Stuffed mushrooms with spinach, cheese, and herbs
147. Tomato and cucumber salad with feta cheese and olives
148. Mini turkey meatballs with marinara sauce
149. Beet and goat cheese crostini
150. Greek yogurt tzatziki with pita triangles
151. Spinach and feta phyllo triangles
152. Cucumber cups filled with crab salad
153. Bell pepper strips with hummus
154. Stuffed cherry tomatoes with herbed goat cheese
155. Smoked salmon pinwheels with cream cheese and dill
156. Grilled shrimp skewers with lemon wedges
157. Guacamole with cucumber slices
158. Stuffed bell peppers with quinoa and black beans
159. Chicken lettuce wraps with lettuce cups and hoisin sauce
160. Greek salad skewers with olives, cucumber, tomato, and feta cheese

161. Baked sweet potato fries with yogurt dipping sauce

162. Turkey roll-ups with cream cheese and spinach leaves

163. Roasted garlic and white bean dip with whole grain crackers

164. Caprese-stuffed portobello mushrooms

165. Buffalo cauliflower bites with Greek yogurt dipping sauce

166. Smoked salmon and avocado salad in cucumber cups

167. Mini vegetable spring rolls with dipping sauce

168. Antipasto platter with olives, cheese, and cured meats

169. Zucchini fritters with yogurt sauce

170. Stuffed jalapeno poppers with cream cheese

171. Tomato bruschetta with basil and garlic on whole grain baguette slices

172. Cucumber slices topped with tuna salad

173. Greek yogurt with sliced strawberries and granola

174. Rice paper rolls with shrimp, vegetables, and dipping sauce

175. Beet hummus with carrot sticks

176. Stuffed cherry peppers with herbed ricotta

177. Bacon-wrapped shrimp with BBQ sauce

178. Roasted cauliflower bites with tahini dipping sauce

179. Stuffed avocado halves with shrimp salad

180. Deviled eggs with avocado instead of mayo

181. Quinoa-stuffed bell peppers with black beans and corn

182. Greek yogurt with mixed berries and honey
183. Artichoke hearts with lemon aioli
184. Zucchini roll-ups with herbed cream cheese
185. Smoked salmon and avocado rolls with cream cheese
186. Bacon-wrapped dates stuffed with almonds
187. Chicken satay skewers with peanut dipping sauce
188. Goat cheese and fig crostini
189. Prosciutto-wrapped melon slices
190. Watermelon and feta skewers with mint
191. Marinated olives with herbs and citrus zest
192. Smoked trout pate on cucumber slices
193. Chicken avocado roll-ups with salsa
194. Buffalo cauliflower bites with blue cheese dipping sauce
195. Crab and avocado stacks with lime dressing
196. Tomato and mozzarella skewers with pesto drizzle
197. Stuffed artichoke hearts with breadcrumbs and Parmesan
198. Cucumber boats filled with Greek yogurt and dill
199. Greek yogurt with sliced peaches and almonds
200. Rice cakes with almond butter and banana slices

These appetizers offer a variety of flavors and textures while being gentle on the digestive system, making them suitable for individuals without a gallbladder. Adjust ingredients and portion sizes according to personal preferences and dietary restrictions.

Healthy Dips and Spreads

Here's healthy dips and spreads suitable for individuals without a gallbladder:

1. Hummus
2. Guacamole
3. Greek yogurt tzatziki
4. Baba ganoush (eggplant dip)
5. White bean dip with garlic and herbs
6. Avocado salsa
7. Spinach and artichoke dip with Greek yogurt
8. Roasted red pepper dip
9. Edamame hummus
10. Beet hummus
11. Cucumber yogurt dip
12. Black bean dip with lime and cilantro
13. Carrot ginger dip
14. Spicy salsa verde
15. Olive tapenade
16. Sun-dried tomato pesto
17. Roasted garlic and herb dip
18. Smoky eggplant dip
19. Lemon dill yogurt dip
20. Jalapeno cilantro hummus
21. Sweet potato hummus
22. Buffalo cauliflower dip
23. Mango avocado salsa
24. Greek yogurt ranch dip

25. Cilantro lime hummus
26. Roasted beet and walnut dip
27. Spicy black bean and corn salsa
28. Greek yogurt onion dip
29. Roasted cauliflower and tahini dip
30. Artichoke and spinach dip
31. Roasted carrot and ginger dip
32. Avocado lime crema
33. Chipotle black bean dip
34. Roasted red pepper and walnut dip
35. Creamy avocado dip with lime and cilantro
36. Smoky sweet potato dip
37. Beet and feta dip
38. Avocado basil pesto
39. Green goddess dip with Greek yogurt
40. Creamy garlic and herb dip
41. Roasted poblano pepper dip
42. Caramelized onion and Greek yogurt dip
43. Spicy avocado salsa
44. Roasted eggplant and red pepper dip
45. Roasted tomato and garlic salsa
46. Cucumber mint yogurt dip
47. Spicy mango salsa
48. Roasted red pepper and feta dip
49. Creamy avocado and black bean dip
50. Cilantro lime Greek yogurt dip
51. Roasted sweet potato and garlic dip
52. Olive and sun-dried tomato tapenade
53. Creamy avocado and lime dip
54. Greek yogurt curry dip
55. Roasted cauliflower and chickpea dip
56. Mango pineapple salsa

57. Roasted garlic and white bean dip
58. Creamy chipotle dip
59. Spicy jalapeno and cilantro hummus
60. Greek yogurt cucumber dill dip
61. Smoky roasted red pepper hummus
62. Creamy avocado and lime crema
63. Roasted poblano and corn salsa
64. Spicy black bean dip with cilantro
65. Creamy feta and spinach dip
66. Avocado cilantro lime dip
67. Roasted butternut squash and garlic dip
68. Greek yogurt buffalo dip
69. Creamy sun-dried tomato and basil dip
70. Chipotle lime Greek yogurt dip
71. Creamy avocado and cucumber dip
72. Roasted carrot and tahini dip
73. Creamy feta and roasted red pepper dip
74. Cilantro lime avocado crema
75. Roasted garlic and chickpea dip
76. Spicy chipotle black bean dip
77. Greek yogurt pesto dip
78. Creamy avocado and black bean salsa
79. Roasted sweet potato and red pepper dip
80. Creamy jalapeno cilantro dip
81. Greek yogurt cucumber mint dip
82. Roasted poblano and avocado salsa
83. Creamy lemon dill yogurt dip
84. Spicy sriracha hummus
85. Creamy avocado and lime salsa
86. Roasted garlic and white bean hummus
87. Chipotle lime black bean dip
88. Creamy feta and olive tapenade

89. Avocado and mango salsa
90. Roasted red pepper and basil hummus
91. Creamy chipotle lime dip
92. Greek yogurt spinach dip
93. Creamy avocado and cilantro lime dip
94. Roasted sweet potato and chickpea dip
95. Creamy sun-dried tomato and basil hummus
96. Cilantro lime black bean dip
97. Greek yogurt curry and turmeric dip
98. Creamy jalapeno and lime dip
99. Roasted cauliflower and garlic hummus
100. Spicy avocado and black bean dip
101. Roasted red pepper and walnut hummus
102. Creamy feta and sun-dried tomato dip
103. Avocado and black bean salsa
104. Roasted garlic and rosemary hummus
105. Greek yogurt tahini dip
106. Creamy avocado and corn salsa
107. Roasted red pepper and garlic dip
108. Chipotle lime avocado dip
109. Creamy feta and roasted garlic dip
110. Greek yogurt harissa dip
111. Creamy jalapeno and cilantro hummus
112. Roasted butternut squash and sage hummus
113. Spicy chipotle lime dip
114. Avocado and black bean hummus
115. Creamy lemon basil yogurt dip
116. Roasted poblano and corn hummus
117. Creamy feta and olive dip
118. Cilantro lime avocado salsa
119. Greek yogurt za'atar dip

Additional Tips:

- Incorporate snacks and appetizers that are rich in fiber to support digestion and keep you feeling full for longer periods.
- Choose lean protein sources like chicken, turkey, fish, and legumes to help meet your protein needs without adding unnecessary fat.
- Be mindful of portion sizes to avoid overeating, especially with snacks and appetizers.
- Stay hydrated throughout the day by drinking water or herbal teas to help aid digestion and prevent dehydration

CHAPTER SIX

Desserts and Sweet Treats

Desserts and sweet treats for individuals without a gallbladder should be low in fat, gentle on the digestive system, and preferably made with ingredients that are easy to tolerate.

Low-Fat Dessert

Here's a list of low-fat dessert ideas suitable for a no gallbladder patient:

1. Fruit salad with honey-lime dressing
2. Mixed berry compote with Greek yogurt
3. Baked apples with cinnamon and raisins
4. Chia seed pudding with fresh fruit
5. Frozen banana slices dipped in dark chocolate
6. Mango sorbet
7. Strawberry banana smoothie popsicles
8. Greek yogurt parfait with granola and berries
9. Poached pears with vanilla yogurt sauce
10. Pineapple sorbet
11. Watermelon slices sprinkled with lime juice
12. Kiwi and strawberry fruit skewers
13. Frozen grapes
14. Peach and raspberry sorbet
15. Rice pudding with almond milk
16. Orange segments drizzled with honey
17. Cantaloupe and honeydew melon balls
18. Frozen yogurt bites

19. Apricot and almond crumble
20. Blueberry and lemon frozen yogurt
21. Grapefruit segments with mint syrup
22. Berry smoothie bowls topped with granola and coconut flakes
23. Raspberry and yogurt popsicles
24. Mixed fruit salsa with cinnamon tortilla chips
25. Baked pear halves with cinnamon and honey
26. Papaya and lime sorbet
27. Grilled pineapple slices with cinnamon
28. Raspberry and coconut chia pudding
29. Mixed fruit kabobs with yogurt dip
30. Strawberry banana yogurt popsicles
31. Fruit salad with mint and lime dressing
32. Plum and almond crumble
33. Mango and pineapple sorbet
34. Peach and blueberry fruit salad
35. Frozen yogurt-covered strawberries
36. Kiwi and mango sorbet
37. Pineapple and coconut chia pudding
38. Orange and vanilla yogurt popsicles
39. Mixed berry crisp with oat topping
40. Watermelon slushies
41. Grilled peach halves with balsamic glaze
42. Frozen banana pops
43. Lemon sorbet
44. Mixed fruit smoothie bowls with shredded coconut
45. Grapefruit and orange segments with honey drizzle
46. Mango and banana frozen yogurt
47. Pineapple and kiwi fruit salsa

48. Honeydew melon and cucumber sorbet
49. Raspberry and peach fruit salad
50. Frozen yogurt-covered blueberries
51. Mixed berry and yogurt parfaits
52. Lemon and raspberry sorbet
53. Kiwi and strawberry sorbet
54. Watermelon and cucumber salad with mint
55. Grilled pineapple and mango skewers
56. Orange and vanilla chia pudding
57. Mango and coconut frozen yogurt
58. Mixed fruit smoothies
59. Grapefruit and pomegranate salad
60. Banana and strawberry fruit salad
61. Berry smoothie bowls with sliced almonds
62. Pineapple and mango salsa
63. Frozen yogurt-covered banana slices
64. Mixed berry and granola parfaits
65. Orange and pineapple sorbet
66. Grapefruit and kiwi fruit salad
67. Berry and yogurt popsicles
68. Kiwi and pineapple sorbet
69. Mango and lime chia pudding
70. Mixed fruit salad with ginger-lime dressing
71. Raspberry and lemon frozen yogurt
72. Grilled pineapple and peach slices
73. Banana and mango sorbet
74. Mixed berry and yogurt popsicles
75. Orange and grapefruit salad with mint
76. Kiwi and raspberry fruit salad
77. Pineapple and banana sorbet
78. Mango and coconut chia pudding
79. Mixed berry smoothie bowls with chia seeds

80. Grilled watermelon wedges with lime
81. Orange and vanilla frozen yogurt
82. Raspberry and almond chia pudding
83. Mango and pineapple fruit salad
84. Frozen grapes dipped in yogurt
85. Mixed berry and yogurt smoothies
86. Kiwi and strawberry fruit salad with basil
87. Pineapple and coconut sorbet
88. Banana and strawberry frozen yogurt
89. Orange and grapefruit sorbet
90. Raspberry and lime chia pudding
91. Mango and banana fruit salad
92. Mixed berry and yogurt smoothie bowls
93. Kiwi and mango fruit salad
94. Pineapple and coconut chia pudding
95. Orange and vanilla yogurt popsicles
96. Raspberry and lime sorbet
97. Mango and banana smoothies
98. Mixed berry and yogurt smoothie popsicles
99. Kiwi and pineapple fruit salad with honey-lime dressing
100. Pineapple and banana smoothie bowls
101. Orange and grapefruit fruit salad with honey-mint dressing
102. Raspberry and coconut chia pudding
103. Mango and banana smoothie popsicles
104. Mixed berry and yogurt popsicles
105. Kiwi and strawberry sorbet
106. Pineapple and coconut yogurt popsicles
107. Orange and vanilla chia pudding
108. Raspberry and lime smoothie bowls
109. Mango and banana sorbet

110. Mixed berry and yogurt smoothies
111. Kiwi and mango chia pudding
112. Pineapple and banana frozen yogurt
113. Orange and grapefruit smoothie bowls
114. Raspberry and coconut smoothies
115. Mango and banana yogurt popsicles
116. Mixed berry and yogurt sorbet
117. Kiwi and pineapple smoothie bowls
118. Pineapple and coconut smoothies
119. Orange and grapefruit yogurt popsicles
120. Raspberry and lime yogurt sorbet
121. Mango and banana smoothie bowls
122. Mixed berry and yogurt chia pudding
123. Kiwi and strawberry smoothies
124. Pineapple and banana yogurt sorbet
125. Orange and grapefruit chia pudding
126. Raspberry and coconut yogurt popsicles
127. Mango and banana chia pudding
128. Mixed berry and yogurt smoothie bowls
129. Kiwi and pineapple yogurt popsicles
130. Pineapple and coconut chia pudding
131. Orange and grapefruit smoothies
132. Raspberry and lime yogurt sorbet
133. Mango and banana yogurt popsicles
134. Mixed berry and yogurt chia pudding
135. Kiwi and strawberry yogurt sorbet
136. Pineapple and banana smoothies
137. Orange and grapefruit yogurt popsicles
138. Raspberry and coconut chia pudding
139. Mango and banana yogurt sorbet
140. Mixed berry and yogurt smoothies
141. Kiwi and pineapple yogurt popsicles

142. Pineapple and coconut smoothie bowls
143. Orange and grapefruit chia pudding
144. Raspberry and lime yogurt popsicles
145. Mango and banana chia pudding
146. Mixed berry and yogurt sorbet
147. Kiwi and strawberry smoothie bowls
148. Pineapple and banana chia pudding
149. Orange and grapefruit yogurt sorbet
150. Raspberry and coconut smoothies
151. Mango and banana yogurt popsicles
152. Mixed berry and yogurt chia pudding
153. Kiwi and pineapple chia pudding
154. Pineapple and coconut yogurt sorbet
155. Orange and grapefruit smoothie bowls
156. Raspberry and lime smoothies
157. Mango and banana yogurt chia pudding
158. Mixed berry and yogurt yogurt popsicles
159. Kiwi and strawberry yogurt sorbet
160. Pineapple and banana smoothie bowls
161. Orange and grapefruit yogurt chia pudding
162. Raspberry and coconut smoothie

Fruit-based desserts

Here's a list of various fruit-based desserts suitable for a no gallbladder patient:

1. Fruit salad with honey-lime dressing
2. Baked apples with cinnamon and raisins
3. Mixed berry compote with Greek yogurt
4. Frozen banana slices dipped in dark chocolate
5. Mango sorbet

6. Strawberry banana smoothie popsicles
7. Poached pears with vanilla yogurt sauce
8. Pineapple sorbet
9. Kiwi and strawberry fruit skewers
10. Frozen grapes
11. Peach and raspberry sorbet
12. Orange segments drizzled with honey
13. Cantaloupe and honeydew melon balls
14. Frozen yogurt bites
15. Apricot and almond crumble
16. Blueberry and lemon frozen yogurt
17. Grapefruit segments with mint syrup
18. Berry smoothie bowls topped with granola and coconut flakes
19. Raspberry and yogurt popsicles
20. Peach and blueberry fruit salad
21. Frozen yogurt-covered strawberries
22. Kiwi and mango sorbet
23. Papaya and lime sorbet
24. Raspberry and coconut chia pudding
25. Mango and pineapple fruit salad
26. Frozen yogurt-covered blueberries
27. Kiwi and raspberry fruit salad
28. Pineapple and coconut chia pudding
29. Orange and vanilla yogurt popsicles
30. Raspberry and lime chia pudding
31. Mango and banana fruit salad
32. Mixed berry and yogurt parfaits
33. Lemon sorbet
34. Mixed berry and yogurt popsicles
35. Kiwi and strawberry sorbet
36. Mango and lime chia pudding

37. Pineapple and coconut yogurt popsicles
38. Raspberry and almond chia pudding
39. Mixed berry and yogurt smoothies
40. Grapefruit and pomegranate salad
41. Banana and strawberry fruit salad
42. Raspberry and coconut smoothie bowls
43. Kiwi and pineapple sorbet
44. Pineapple and banana sorbet
45. Mango and banana yogurt popsicles
46. Mixed berry and yogurt sorbet
47. Kiwi and strawberry smoothies
48. Raspberry and lime smoothie bowls
49. Mango and banana chia pudding
50. Pineapple and coconut smoothie bowls
51. Raspberry and coconut yogurt popsicles
52. Kiwi and pineapple smoothie bowls
53. Orange and grapefruit yogurt popsicles
54. Mango and banana yogurt chia pudding
55. Mixed berry and yogurt yogurt popsicles
56. Pineapple and banana smoothie bowls
57. Raspberry and lime yogurt popsicles
58. Mango and banana smoothie bowls
59. Kiwi and strawberry yogurt sorbet
60. Orange and grapefruit smoothie bowls
61. Raspberry and coconut smoothies
62. Mango and banana chia pudding
63. Pineapple and coconut yogurt sorbet
64. Kiwi and mango smoothie bowls
65. Orange and grapefruit yogurt chia pudding
66. Raspberry and lime sorbet
67. Mango and banana smoothies
68. Kiwi and pineapple yogurt popsicles

69. Pineapple and coconut chia pudding
70. Orange and grapefruit sorbet
71. Raspberry and almond yogurt popsicles
72. Mango and banana yogurt sorbet
73. Kiwi and strawberry smoothie bowls
74. Pineapple and banana chia pudding
75. Orange and vanilla yogurt popsicles
76. Raspberry and lime chia pudding
77. Mango and banana smoothies
78. Kiwi and mango chia pudding
79. Orange and grapefruit smoothie bowls
80. Raspberry and coconut yogurt popsicles
81. Mango and banana chia pudding
82. Mixed berry and yogurt yogurt popsicles
83. Kiwi and pineapple chia pudding
84. Pineapple and coconut yogurt sorbet
85. Orange and grapefruit smoothie bowls
86. Raspberry and lime smoothies
87. Mango and banana yogurt chia pudding
88. Kiwi and strawberry yogurt sorbet
89. Pineapple and banana smoothie bowls
90. Orange and grapefruit yogurt chia pudding
91. Raspberry and coconut smoothies
92. Mango and banana yogurt popsicles
93. Kiwi and pineapple yogurt sorbet
94. Pineapple and coconut chia pudding
95. Orange and grapefruit sorbet
96. Raspberry and almond chia pudding
97. Mango and banana smoothie bowls
98. Kiwi and strawberry smoothies
99. Pineapple and banana yogurt popsicles
100. Orange and grapefruit smoothie bowls

101. Raspberry and lime sorbet
102. Mango and banana chia pudding
103. Kiwi and pineapple smoothie bowls
104. Pineapple and coconut smoothies
105. Orange and grapefruit yogurt popsicles
106. Raspberry and coconut yogurt popsicles
107. Mango and banana yogurt chia pudding
108. Kiwi and strawberry yogurt sorbet
109. Pineapple and banana chia pudding
110. Orange and vanilla yogurt popsicles
111. Raspberry and lime yogurt sorbet
112. Mango and banana smoothie bowls
113. Kiwi and mango yogurt popsicles
114. Pineapple and coconut chia pudding
115. Orange and grapefruit sorbet
116. Raspberry and coconut chia pudding
117. Mango and banana yogurt sorbet
118. Kiwi and strawberry smoothie bowls
119. Pineapple and banana chia pudding
120. Orange and grapefruit yogurt chia pudding
121. Raspberry and lime smoothie bowls
122. Mango and banana chia pudding
123. Kiwi and pineapple chia pudding

Additional Tips:

- Use natural sweeteners like honey, maple syrup, or stevia instead of refined sugars to sweeten desserts.

- Experiment with spices like cinnamon, nutmeg, or ginger to add flavor without adding extra fat.

- Incorporate small portions of desserts and sweet treats into your overall diet to enjoy without overloading your system.
- Listen to your body and pay attention to how different ingredients affect your digestion to find the most suitable options for you.

These dessert ideas offer delicious and satisfying treats for individuals without a gallbladder while keeping dietary needs and digestive comfort in mind. Enjoy these sweet treats in moderation as part of a balanced and healthy diet.

Baking Substitutions for Healthier Options

Baking substitutions for individuals without a gallbladder aim to reduce fat content, incorporate healthier options, and ensure ease of digestion.

Here are some baking substitutions for healthier options:

1. Applesauce: Substitute applesauce for oil or butter in recipes like cakes, muffins, and bread to reduce fat content.

2. Greek Yogurt: Replace sour cream or mayonnaise with Greek yogurt in recipes for added protein and reduced fat.

3. Avocado: Use mashed avocado as a substitute for butter in recipes like brownies or cookies for a healthier fat alternative.

4. Coconut Oil: Substitute coconut oil for butter or vegetable oil in baking recipes for a healthier fat option.

5. Almond Flour: Replace all-purpose flour with almond flour in recipes to increase protein and reduce carbohydrates.

6. Oat Flour: Use oat flour instead of traditional flour for a higher fiber content and a gluten-free option.

7. Bananas: Use mashed ripe bananas as a natural sweetener and binder in recipes like pancakes, muffins, and cookies.

8. Honey or Maple Syrup: Replace granulated sugar with honey or maple syrup for natural sweetness and added flavor.

9. Almond Milk: Substitute almond milk for regular milk in recipes to reduce lactose intake and lower fat content.

10. Flaxseed Meal: Use flaxseed meal mixed with water as an egg substitute in recipes for binding properties and omega-3 fatty acids.

11. Unsweetened Cocoa Powder: Opt for unsweetened cocoa powder instead of chocolate chips or cocoa mixes to reduce added sugars.

12. Nut Butters: Use natural nut butters like almond butter or peanut butter as a spread or ingredient in baking for healthier fats.

13. Coconut Sugar: Substitute coconut sugar for white or brown sugar as a lower glycemic index alternative.

14. Stevia: Use stevia as a zero-calorie sweetener option in baking recipes to reduce sugar intake.

15. Whole Wheat Flour: Replace refined white flour with whole wheat flour for added fiber and nutrients in baked goods.

16. Mashed Sweet Potatoes: Incorporate mashed sweet potatoes into recipes like muffins or bread for natural sweetness and moisture.

17. Chia Seeds: Use chia seeds mixed with water as an egg substitute for binding and nutritional benefits.

18. Prune Puree: Replace fats like butter or oil with prune puree for added moisture and natural sweetness in baked goods.

19. Non-Dairy Yogurt: Substitute non-dairy yogurt like coconut or almond yogurt for dairy-based yogurt in recipes for lactose-free options.

20. Quinoa Flour: Use quinoa flour instead of traditional flour for a gluten-free option with added protein and nutrients.

Tips:

- Experiment with different substitutions to find the ones that work best for your taste preferences and dietary needs.
- Pay attention to portion sizes and overall calorie intake, even with healthier substitutions.
- Gradually introduce substitutions to your recipes to adjust to new flavors and textures.

- Read labels carefully to ensure that substituted ingredients are free of additives, preservatives, and other ingredients that may cause discomfort.

These substitutions can help make baked goods healthier and more suitable for individuals without a gallbladder, while still maintaining flavor and texture. Adjust quantities and ingredients according to personal preferences and dietary restrictions.

CHAPTER SEVEN

Beverages and Hydration

Beverages and hydration are crucial aspects of maintaining overall health and well-being, especially for individuals without a gallbladder. Proper hydration supports digestion, helps regulate body temperature, and facilitates the transport of nutrients throughout the body.

Hydration Importance After Gallbladder Removal"

Hydration importance after gallbladder removal, also known as cholecystectomy, cannot be overstated. The gallbladder is an organ that stores bile produced by the liver, aiding in the digestion of fats. After gallbladder removal, bile flows directly from the liver into the small intestine, which can impact digestion and nutrient absorption. Here's why hydration is crucial after gallbladder removal:

1. Digestive Support:
   Hydration helps to soften stools and promote regular bowel movements, which can alleviate constipation, a common issue after gallbladder removal.

2. Bile Production and Function:

Adequate hydration supports the production and flow of bile from the liver to the small intestine. Bile helps emulsify fats and aids in their digestion, compensating for the absence of the gallbladder.

3. Nutrient Absorption:

Hydration plays a key role in facilitating the absorption of nutrients, including fat-soluble vitamins like A, D, E, and K, which are essential for various bodily functions.

4. Prevention of Bile Duct Complications:

Dehydration can lead to the thickening of bile, increasing the risk of bile duct complications such as bile duct stones or inflammation.

5. Alleviation of Digestive Discomfort:

Proper hydration can help alleviate digestive discomfort, bloating, and gas, which may occur as the body adjusts to the absence of the gallbladder.

Tips for Hydration After Gallbladder Removal:

1. Drink Plenty of Water: Aim to drink at least 8 glasses of water per day, or more if you're physically active or live in a hot climate. Sip water throughout the day rather than consuming large amounts at once.

2. Consider Electrolyte Balance: In addition to water, consider beverages or foods that contain electrolytes, such as coconut water or electrolyte solutions, especially if you experience diarrhea or excessive sweating.

3. Limit Caffeine and Alcohol: Caffeinated and alcoholic beverages can contribute to dehydration, so consume them in moderation and balance with water intake.

4. Monitor Urine Color: Aim for pale yellow urine, which indicates adequate hydration. Dark yellow urine may indicate dehydration.

5. Hydrate Before, During, and After Meals: Drink water before, during, and after meals to aid digestion and promote the flow of bile into the small intestine.

6. Include Hydrating Foods: Incorporate hydrating foods like fruits and vegetables into your diet, which contribute to overall hydration levels.

Consult Your Healthcare Provider:
If you experience persistent dehydration, digestive discomfort, or changes in bowel habits after gallbladder removal, consult your healthcare provider. They can offer personalized recommendations and ensure that you're adequately hydrated while managing any digestive issues effectively. Prioritizing hydration is essential

for supporting digestion, nutrient absorption, and overall well-being after gallbladder removal.

Low-Sugar Drink Choices

Low-sugar drink choices are essential for maintaining overall health, managing blood sugar levels, and reducing the risk of chronic diseases such as obesity, diabetes, and cardiovascular conditions. Here are some options for low-sugar drinks:

1. Water:

Plain water is the healthiest and most hydrating option available. It contains zero calories and no added sugars, making it the perfect choice for quenching thirst without impacting blood sugar levels.

2. Herbal Teas:

Herbal teas like chamomile, peppermint, ginger, and rooibos are naturally caffeine-free and sugar-free. They offer a variety of flavors and can be enjoyed hot or cold.

3. Green Tea:

Green tea is rich in antioxidants and contains minimal calories and sugar when consumed without added sweeteners. It provides a gentle energy boost and may offer various health benefits.

4. Sparkling Water:

Sparkling water, whether plain or flavored with natural essences, provides the refreshing fizz of soda without the added sugars or calories. It can be a satisfying alternative to sugary sodas and soft drinks.

5. Infused Water:

Infused water is made by adding fruits, vegetables, and herbs to plain water to infuse it with flavor. Popular combinations include cucumber and mint, lemon and ginger, or berries and basil.

6. Unsweetened Almond Milk or Coconut Milk:

Unsweetened almond milk or coconut milk is a dairy-free and low-calorie alternative to cow's milk. Choose unsweetened varieties to minimize sugar intake.

7. Vegetable Juices:

Vegetable juices, such as tomato, cucumber, or celery juice, are naturally low in sugar and calories while providing essential vitamins, minerals, and antioxidants.

8. Homemade Smoothies:

Prepare homemade smoothies using low-sugar fruits like berries, avocado, and citrus fruits. Add leafy greens like spinach or kale for extra nutrients and fiber.

9. Iced Herbal Lemonades:

Make refreshing herbal lemonades by combining freshly squeezed lemon juice with water and sweetening lightly with stevia or a small amount of honey or maple syrup.

10. Cold Brew Coffee:

Cold brew coffee is naturally lower in acidity and bitterness compared to hot brewed coffee. Enjoy it plain or with a splash of unsweetened almond milk for a low-sugar caffeinated beverage.

Tips for Choosing Low-Sugar Drinks:

- Read labels carefully to identify hidden sugars in beverages, including natural sweeteners like honey, agave syrup, and fruit juice concentrates.
- Opt for beverages with no added sugars or choose those sweetened with natural sweeteners like stevia or monk fruit extract.
- Be mindful of portion sizes and avoid consuming large quantities of even low-sugar beverages, especially if managing blood sugar levels or weight.

Choosing low-sugar drink options can help promote hydration, support overall health, and contribute to a balanced diet without compromising on flavor or enjoyment.

Herbal Teas and Infusions

Herbal teas and infusions are popular beverages known for their soothing flavors, aromatic profiles, and potential health benefits. Unlike traditional tea, which comes from the Camellia sinensis plant, herbal teas are made from dried fruits, flowers, herbs, and spices. Here's an overview of herbal teas and infusions:

Types of Herbal Teas:

1. Chamomile Tea:

Chamomile tea is well-known for its calming properties and mild, floral flavor. It is often consumed before bedtime to promote relaxation and improve sleep quality.

2. Peppermint Tea:

Peppermint tea has a refreshing and invigorating flavor, with natural menthol providing a cooling sensation. It is commonly used to aid digestion, alleviate nausea, and relieve headaches.

3. Ginger Tea:

Ginger tea is made from fresh or dried ginger root and has a spicy, warming flavor. It is praised for its anti-inflammatory properties and digestive benefits, making it a popular choice after meals.

4. Lemon Balm Tea:

Lemon balm tea has a mild, lemony flavor and is known for its calming effects on the nervous system. It may help reduce anxiety, improve mood, and promote relaxation.

5. Hibiscus Tea:

Hibiscus tea is made from the dried petals of the hibiscus flower and has a tart, cranberry-like flavor. It is rich in antioxidants and may help lower blood pressure and improve heart health.

6. Lavender Tea:

Lavender tea has a delicate floral aroma and is prized for its relaxing and stress-relieving properties. It is often used to promote relaxation and improve sleep quality.

Benefits of Herbal Teas and Infusions:

Promotes Hydration: Herbal teas are hydrating and can contribute to your daily fluid intake, making them a healthy alternative to sugary beverages.

Supports Digestive Health: Many herbal teas, such as ginger and peppermint, have been traditionally used to aid digestion, alleviate bloating, and relieve gastrointestinal discomfort.

Provides Antioxidants: Herbal teas are rich in antioxidants, which help protect cells from damage caused by free radicals and may reduce the risk of chronic diseases.

Encourages Relaxation: Certain herbal teas, like chamomile and lemon balm, have calming properties that can help reduce stress, anxiety, and promote relaxation.

Brewing Herbal Teas and Infusions:

Water Temperature: Herbal teas are typically brewed with boiling water, but delicate herbs like chamomile may benefit from slightly cooler water to preserve their delicate flavors.

Steeping Time: Steep herbal teas for 5-10 minutes to extract their flavors and health benefits fully. Longer steeping times may result in a stronger, more pronounced flavor.

Sweeteners and Enhancements: Herbal teas can be enjoyed plain or sweetened with honey, maple syrup, or a splash of lemon juice. Experiment with additions like fresh ginger, cinnamon sticks, or citrus peels to customize your brew.

Herbal teas and infusions offer a delightful array of flavors, aromas, and potential health benefits. Whether you're seeking relaxation, digestive support, or simply a flavorful beverage, there's a herbal tea to suit every palate and occasion. Incorporate herbal teas into your daily routine to enjoy their soothing effects and nourishing properties.

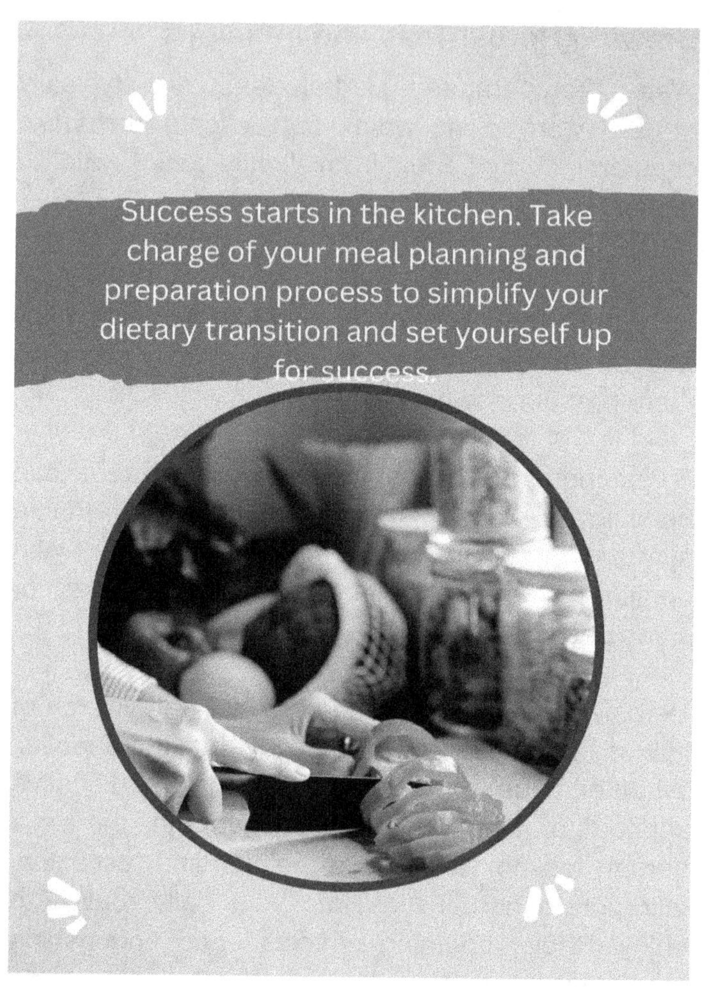

Success starts in the kitchen. Take charge of your meal planning and preparation process to simplify your dietary transition and set yourself up for success.

CHAPTER EIGHT

Lifestyle and Wellness Tips

Living a healthy lifestyle after gallbladder removal involves incorporating physical activity, managing stress effectively, and tracking dietary changes and symptoms. Here's a comprehensive guide on lifestyle and wellness tips for individuals without a gallbladder:

1. Incorporating Physical Activity:

Start Slowly: Begin with low-impact activities such as walking, swimming, or yoga, and gradually increase intensity and duration as tolerated.

Find Enjoyable Activities: Choose activities that you enjoy and are sustainable for the long term. This could include dancing, hiking, cycling, or participating in group fitness classes.

Be Consistent: Aim for at least 150 minutes of moderate-intensity aerobic activity or 75 minutes of vigorous-intensity aerobic activity per week, spread throughout the week.

Include Strength Training: Incorporate strength training exercises at least two days per week to build muscle mass, improve metabolism, and support overall health.

2. **Stress Management Techniques**:

Practice Mindfulness: Engage in mindfulness meditation, deep breathing exercises, or progressive muscle relaxation to reduce stress levels and promote relaxation.

Prioritize Self-Care: Make time for activities that nourish your mind, body, and soul, such as spending time in nature, reading, listening to music, or pursuing hobbies.

Establish Boundaries: Learn to say no to commitments or activities that cause unnecessary stress and prioritize activities that align with your values and priorities.

Seek Support: Reach out to friends, family members, or support groups for emotional support and encouragement during challenging times.

3. **Tracking Dietary Changes and Symptoms:**

Keep a Food Diary: Maintain a food diary to track your dietary intake, including meals, snacks, portion sizes, and any symptoms experienced after eating.

Monitor Symptoms: Pay attention to how your body responds to different foods and beverages. Note any digestive symptoms such as bloating, gas, diarrhea, or abdominal discomfort.

Identify Triggers: Identify foods or beverages that may trigger digestive discomfort or symptoms and consider eliminating or reducing them from your diet.

Consult a Registered Dietitian: Seek guidance from a registered dietitian who can help you develop a personalized eating plan tailored to your nutritional needs, digestive health, and dietary preferences.

Gradual Dietary Changes: Make gradual dietary changes and observe how your body responds over time. Be patient and flexible as you navigate dietary adjustments post-gallbladder removal.

Additional Tips:

Stay hydrated by drinking plenty of water throughout the day, as hydration is essential for digestion and overall health.

Practice portion control and mindful eating to prevent overeating and promote satiety.

Aim for a balanced diet rich in fruits, vegetables, whole grains, lean proteins, and healthy fats to support optimal health and well-being.

Listen to your body's hunger and fullness cues, and eat intuitively rather than relying on external cues or restrictive eating patterns.

By incorporating physical activity, stress management techniques, and mindful dietary practices, individuals without a gallbladder can support their overall health and well-being while managing digestive symptoms and promoting optimal digestion and nutrient absorption. It's important to consult with healthcare professionals for personalized guidance and support along your wellness journey.

CONCLUSION

Living well without a gallbladder requires a combination of dietary modifications, lifestyle adjustments, and self-care practices. While the absence of the gallbladder may present challenges, it's entirely possible to lead a fulfilling and healthy life by making informed choices and prioritizing your well-being.

Final Thoughts on Living Well Without a Gallbladder:

Embrace Adaptation: Adjusting to life without a gallbladder may take time, patience, and experimentation. Be open to trying new foods, lifestyle changes, and wellness practices to find what works best for you.

Listen to Your Body: Pay attention to your body's signals and responses to different foods, activities, and stressors. Tune into your body's cues and make adjustments accordingly to support optimal digestion and overall health.

Seek Support and Guidance: Don't hesitate to reach out to healthcare professionals, registered dietitians, or support groups for guidance, encouragement, and practical tips for managing life without a gallbladder.

Encouragement and Support for Dietary Success:

Celebrate Progress: Celebrate your successes, no matter how small, along your journey toward optimal health and well-being. Recognize the efforts you're making to prioritize your health and take pride in your accomplishments.

Stay Positive: Maintain a positive mindset and outlook, even in the face of challenges or setbacks. Approach dietary changes and lifestyle adjustments with curiosity, resilience, and determination.

Practice Self-Compassion: Be kind to yourself as you navigate dietary changes, symptom management, and lifestyle adjustments. Embrace self-compassion and forgive yourself for any perceived missteps or deviations from your wellness goals.

Stay Connected: Surround yourself with supportive friends, family members, or peers who understand your journey and can provide encouragement, empathy, and accountability along the way.

Living well without a gallbladder is about empowering yourself to make informed choices, prioritize self-care, and cultivate a sense of resilience and well-being. With dedication, patience, and support, you can navigate dietary challenges, embrace lifestyle adjustments, and thrive in your journey toward optimal health and vitality. Remember, you're not alone, and every step you take toward wellness is a step toward living your best life.

Appendix

Glossary of Terms:

Bile is a digestive juice that the liver produces and the gallbladder stores. Aids in the digesting process by breaking down lipids.

Cholecystectomy: Surgical removal of the gallbladder.

Digestive Enzymes: Substances produced by the body to aid in the digestion and absorption of nutrients from food.

Gallstones: Hardened deposits that form in the gallbladder, often composed of cholesterol, bile salts, and calcium salts.

Hydration: The process of maintaining adequate fluid levels in the body to support various physiological functions.

Nutrient Absorption: The process by which nutrients from food are absorbed into the bloodstream and transported to cells throughout the body for energy and growth.

Sample Shopping Lists:

1. Fresh Produce:
   - Leafy greens (spinach, kale, lettuce)

- Berries (blueberries, strawberries, raspberries)
- Citrus fruits (lemons, oranges, grapefruits)
- Avocados
- Tomatoes
- Cucumbers
- Bell peppers
- Apples
- Bananas

2. Proteins:
   - Lean meats (chicken breast, turkey, fish)
   - Eggs
   - Tofu
   - Legumes (beans, lentils, chickpeas)
   - Dairy goods low in fat (like Greek yogurt and cottage cheese)

3. Grains and Legumes:
   - Whole grain bread
   - Quinoa
   - Brown rice
   - Oats
   - Whole wheat pasta
   - Barley

4. Healthy Fats:
   - Olive oil
   - Avocado oil
   - Nuts (almonds, walnuts, pistachios)
   - Seeds: flaxseeds, pumpkin seeds, chia seeds

5. Dairy and Alternatives:

- Low-fat milk or plant-based milk (almond milk, coconut milk)
  - Low-fat cheese
  - Soy milk or yogurt

6. Herbs, Spices, and Condiments:
  - Garlic
  - Ginger
  - Turmeric
  - Cinnamon
  - Herbs (parsley, basil, cilantro)
  - Vinegar (apple cider vinegar, balsamic vinegar)
  - Low-sodium soy sauce

Conversion Charts:

- Liquid Measurements:
  - 8 fluid ounces times one cup is 240 milliliters.
  - 1 tablespoon = 0.5 fluid ounces = 15 milliliters
  - 1 teaspoon = 0.17 fluid ounces = 5 milliliters

- Dry Measurements:
  - 1 cup = 8 ounces = 240 grams
  - 1 tablespoon = 0.5 ounces = 15 grams
  - 1 teaspoon = 0.17 ounces = 5 grams

- Temperature Conversion:
  - Celsius to Fahrenheit: °F = (°C × 9/5) + 32
  - Fahrenheit to Celsius: °C = (°F - 32) × 5/9

These conversion charts and sample shopping lists are designed to assist you in meal planning, grocery shopping, and cooking for your no gallbladder diet. Use them as references to create delicious and nutritious meals tailored to your dietary needs and preferences.

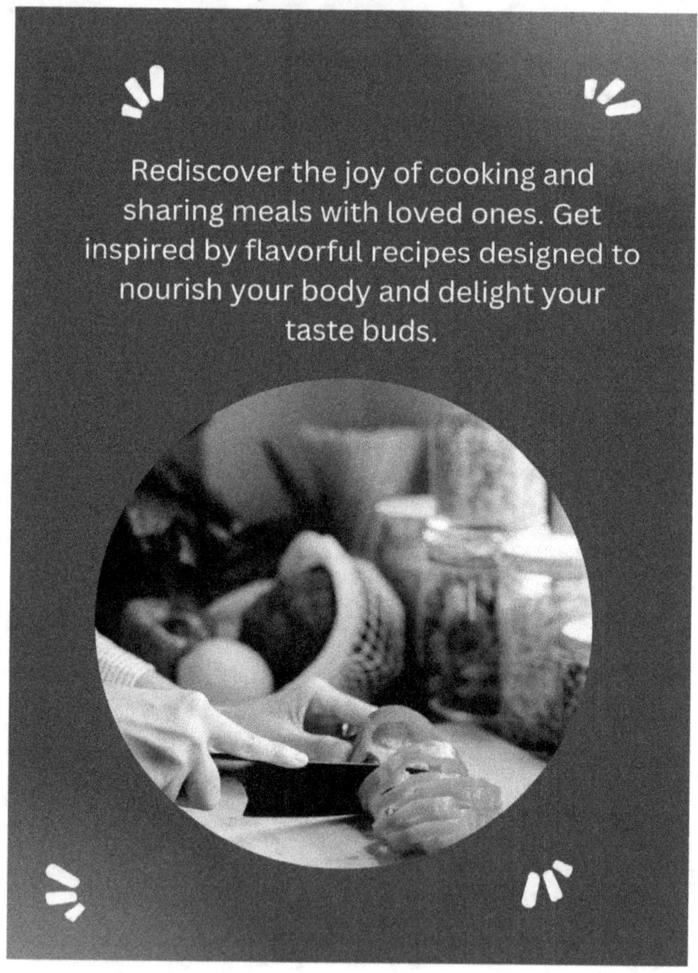

Bonus

30-day Sample Meal Plan

A 30-day sample meal plan for a patient without a gallbladder:

Day 1:
- Breakfast: Scrambled eggs with spinach and avocado
- Lunch consists of grilled chicken salad dressed with balsamic vinaigrette, mixed greens, and cherry tomatoes.
- Dinner: Baked salmon with roasted asparagus and quinoa
- Snack: Greek yogurt with berries

Day 2:
  Almond milk, sliced almonds, chia seeds, and oatmeal for breakfast
  Lunch is lettuce wraps with turkey and avocado with carrot sticks on the side.
Dinner is stuffed bell peppers with quinoa and served with a side salad. Snack is almond butter-topped apple slices.

Day 3:
  Breakfast consists of a spinach, banana, almond milk, and protein powder scoop added to a green smoothie.

Lunch: Lentil soup with a side of mixed greens salad.

Dinner: Grilled chicken breast with steamed broccoli and brown rice;

Snack: Celery sticks with hummus;

Day 4:
- Greek yogurt with mixed berries and granola for breakfast
- Quinoa salad with black beans and grilled shrimp for lunch
Snack: Mixed nuts; Dinner: Baked cod with roasted sweet potatoes and green beans

Day 5:
- Breakfast: Gluten-free pancakes with fresh fruit and a drizzle of maple syrup
- Lunch: Chicken Caesar salad with homemade dressing
- Dinner is marinara sauced baked turkey meatballs paired with zucchini pasta.
- Snack: Carrot sticks with tzatziki dip

Day 6:
- Breakfast: Vegetable omelette with feta cheese
- Lunch: Quinoa and roasted vegetable salad
- Dinner is tomato sauce, zucchini noodles, and grilled shrimp.
- Snack: Hard-boiled eggs

Day 7:

- Breakfast: Chia seed pudding made with almond milk and topped with sliced almonds and berries
- Lunch: Spinach salad with grilled chicken, cherry tomatoes, and avocado
- Dinner: Baked cod with mango salsa and quinoa
- Snack: Edamame beans

Day 8:
- Breakfast: Berry smoothie bowl with spinach, almond milk, and a variety of toppings like granola and sliced fruit
- Lunch would be a lettuce and tomato wrap with turkey and avocado.
- Dinner: Grilled chicken with sweet potato fries and a side salad
- Snack: Rice cakes with almond butter

Day 9:
- Breakfast: Quinoa porridge with almond butter, sliced bananas, and a sprinkle of cinnamon
- Lunch: Chickpea salad with lemon dressing
- Supper is baked salmon paired with roasted veggies and quinoa.
- Snack: Greek yogurt with honey

Day 10:
- Breakfast: Egg muffins with vegetables and cheese
- Lunch would be quinoa, roasted veggies, and grilled chicken.
- Dinner: Baked turkey breast with cauliflower rice and steamed asparagus

- Snack: Carrot and cucumber slices with hummus.

Day 11:
- Breakfast: Green smoothie with spinach, banana, almond milk, and a scoop of protein powder
- Lunch: Lentil curry with brown rice and a side of steamed broccoli
- Dinner: Baked cod with roasted Brussels sprouts and quinoa
- Snack: Carrot sticks with hummus

Day 12:
- Breakfast: Veggie omelette with mushrooms, bell peppers, and goat cheese
- Lunch: Quinoa and black bean burger with lettuce, tomato, and avocado
- Dinner is roasted sweet potatoes, green beans, and grilled chicken breast.
- Snack: Mixed nuts

Day 13:
- Breakfast: Overnight oats with almond milk, chia seeds, and a mix of berries
- Lunch: Greek salad with grilled shrimp and a side of whole grain pita bread
- Dinner: Baked salmon with quinoa and roasted asparagus
- Snack: Apple slices with almond butter

Day 14:
- Breakfast: Gluten-free pancakes with fresh fruit and a drizzle of honey

- Lunch: Chicken Caesar wrap with lettuce, tomato, and Caesar dressing
- Dinner is marinara sauce and baked turkey meatballs with zucchini pasta.
- Snack: mixed berries, granola, and Greek yogurt

Day 15:
- Breakfast: Chia seed pudding made with almond milk and topped with sliced almonds and diced mango
- Lunch: Spinach and quinoa salad with grilled chicken, cherry tomatoes, and balsamic vinaigrette
- Dinner: Grilled shrimp skewers with quinoa and roasted sweet potatoes
- Snack: Rice cakes with almond butter

Day 16:
- Breakfast: Berry smoothie bowl with spinach, almond milk, and a variety of toppings like granola and sliced fruit
- Lunch is lettuce wraps with turkey and avocado and carrot sticks on the side.
- Dinner: Baked cod with mango salsa, brown rice, and steamed asparagus
- Snack: Hard-boiled eggs

Day 17:
- Breakfast: Vegetable omelette with feta cheese and a side of whole grain toast
- Lunch: Quinoa and roasted vegetable salad with grilled chicken

- Dinner: Baked chicken breast with cauliflower rice and roasted broccoli
- Snack: Edamame beans

Day 18:
- Breakfast: Quinoa porridge with almond butter, sliced bananas, and a sprinkle of cinnamon
- Lunch: Chickpea salad with lemon dressing and a side of mixed greens
- Supper is baked salmon paired with roasted veggies and quinoa.
- Snack: Greek yogurt with honey and crushed walnuts

Day 19:
- Breakfast: Scrambled eggs with sautéed spinach and tomatoes
- Lunch: Greek salad with grilled chicken, cucumber, olives, and feta cheese
- Dinner: Grilled shrimp skewers with quinoa and steamed asparagus
- Snack: Carrot sticks with tzatziki dip

Day 20:
- Breakfast: Green smoothie with spinach, banana, almond milk, and a scoop of protein powder
- Lunch would be a mixed green salad on the side and lentil soup.
- Dinner: Baked cod with quinoa and roasted Brussels sprouts
- Snack: Mixed nuts

Day 21:
- Breakfast: Oatmeal with almond milk, sliced almonds, and diced apples
- Lunch consists of grilled chicken salad topped with cherry tomatoes, mixed greens, and balsamic vinaigrette.
- Dinner: Baked salmon with roasted asparagus and quinoa
- Snack: Greek yogurt with berries

Day 22:
- Breakfast: Vegetable omelette with mushrooms, bell peppers, and goat cheese
- Lunch: Turkey and avocado wrap with lettuce, tomato, and mustard
- Dinner: Baked turkey breast with cauliflower rice and steamed broccoli
- Snack: Carrot sticks with hummus

Day 23:
- Breakfast: Chia seed pudding made with almond milk, topped with sliced almonds and diced peaches
- Lunch: Lentil curry with brown rice and a side of steamed spinach
- Dinner is roasted sweet potatoes, green beans, and grilled chicken breast.
- Snack: Mixed nuts

Day 24:
- Breakfast: Gluten-free pancakes with fresh fruit and a drizzle of maple syrup

- Lunch: Quinoa and black bean salad with grilled shrimp
- Dinner: Baked cod with roasted Brussels sprouts and quinoa
- Snack: Apple slices with almond butter

Day 25:
- Breakfast: Green smoothie with spinach, banana, almond milk, and a scoop of protein powder
- Lunch: Chicken Caesar salad with homemade dressing and a side of whole grain pita bread
- Dinner: Baked turkey meatballs with zucchini noodles and marinara sauce
- Snack: Greek yogurt with granola and mixed berries

Day 26:
- Breakfast consists of an omelette made with vegetables, tomatoes, and feta cheese.
- Quinoa-stuffed bell peppers and a side salad for lunch
- Dinner is tomato sauce, zucchini noodles, and grilled shrimp.
- Snack: Almond butter-topped rice cakes

Day 27:
- Breakfast: Berry smoothie bowl with spinach, almond milk, and a variety of toppings like granola and sliced fruit
- Lunch is lettuce wraps with turkey and avocado and carrot sticks on the side.

- Dinner: Baked cod with mango salsa, brown rice, and steamed asparagus
- Snack: Hard-boiled eggs

Day 28:
- Breakfast: Quinoa porridge with almond butter, sliced bananas, and a sprinkle of cinnamon
- Lunch: Chickpea salad with lemon dressing and a side of mixed greens
- Supper is baked salmon paired with roasted veggies and quinoa.
- Snack: Greek yogurt with honey and crushed walnuts

Day 29:
- Breakfast: Scrambled eggs with sautéed spinach and tomatoes
- Lunch would be a mixed green salad on the side and lentil soup.
- Dinner is roasted sweet potatoes and green beans along with grilled chicken breast.
- Snack: Carrot sticks with tzatziki dip

Day 30:
- Breakfast: Green smoothie with spinach, banana, almond milk, and a scoop of protein powder
- Lunch: Quinoa and roasted vegetable salad with grilled chicken
- Dinner: Baked chicken breast with cauliflower rice and roasted broccoli
- Snack: Edamame beans

Remember to adjust portion sizes and ingredients based on the individual's preferences and dietary needs, ensuring a variety of proteins, vegetables, healthy fats, and complex carbohydrates.

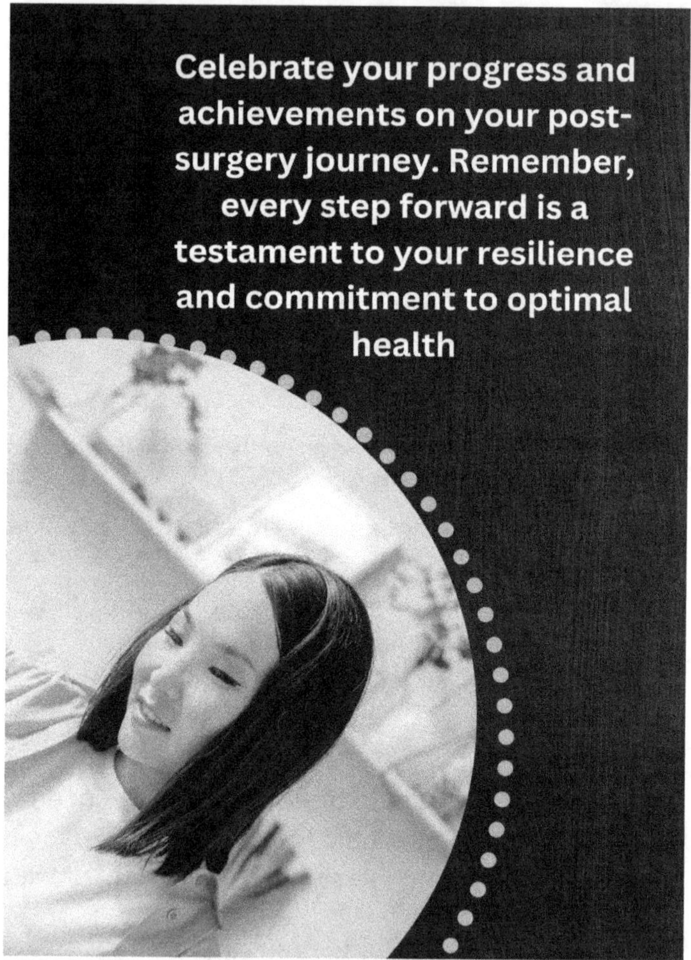